The Lean Body Promise

Your Future Body:
an Owner's Manual

Dr. Vince Quas

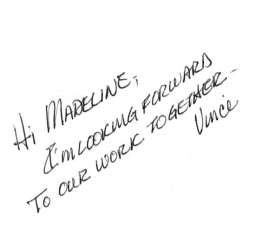
First Edition

Synesis Press, Bend, Oregon

The Lean Body Promise

Your Future Body:
an Owner's Manual

by Dr. Vince Quas

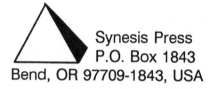

Synesis Press
P.O. Box 1843
Bend, OR 97709-1843, USA

Library of Congress Cataloging In Publication Data

Quas, Vince Dr.
  The Lean Body Promise
  Your Future Body: an Owner's Manual
  Bibliography: p.
1. Reducing diets.   2. Reducing exercises.
3. Body image.   I Title.
RM222.2.Q37   1989   613.2'5--dc19   89-4162
ISBN 0-925572-36-5   ($15.95)

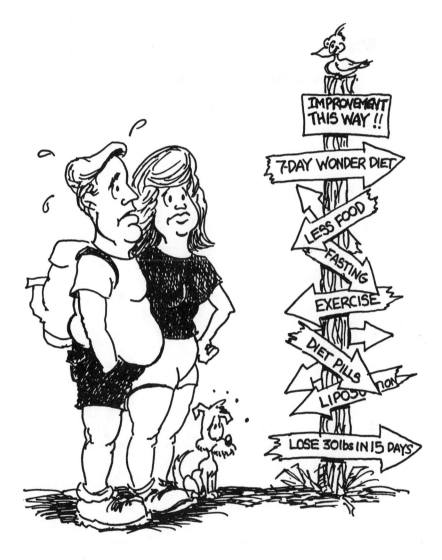

**Perhaps, there is one direction that will solve
the mystery of weight and shape control.**

When we take away our self-imposed

beliefs, excuses and reasons,

all that is left is action.

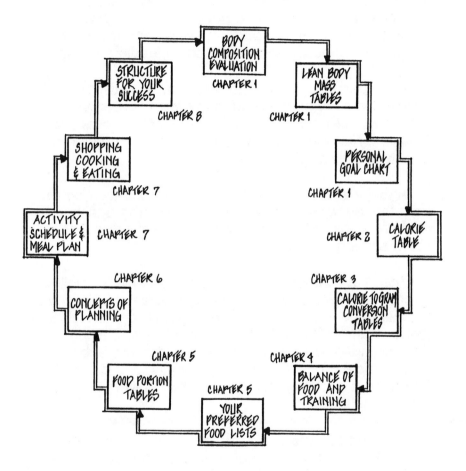

BODY COMPOSITION EVALUATION
CHAPTER 1

STRUCTURE FOR YOUR SUCCESS
CHAPTER 8

LEAN BODY MASS TABLES
CHAPTER 1

SHOPPING COOKING & EATING
CHAPTER 7

PERSONAL GOAL CHART
CHAPTER 1

ACTIVITY SCHEDULE & MEAL PLAN
CHAPTER 7

CALORIE TABLE
CHAPTER 2

CONCEPTS OF PLANNING
CHAPTER 6

CALORIE TO GRAM CONVERSION TABLES
CHAPTER 3

FOOD PORTION TABLES
CHAPTER 5

YOUR PREFERRED FOOD LISTS
CHAPTER 5

BALANCE OF FOOD AND TRAINING
CHAPTER 4

Acknowledgments

Taking inventory of who to acknowledge for their contribution and encouragement was a truly rewarding experience. It helps me realize how seldom I stop to thank those who teach and support me daily, and those who shaped my curiosity and approach by leading the way.

An expanding group of family, friends, patients and colleagues have participated in this work, experienced great improvement and, in essence, have become my teachers. Many who first were teachers, have become friends and extended family.

A major source of my learning and inspiration comes from the following unique blend of people who, although different in their styles, messages and technology, share these same qualities:

They have taken on the challenge and responsibility of contributing to others by being the example. They are teachers and leaders who, by demonstration, stretch and test our perception of limits, performance and aging. They are visionaries who question our traditional beliefs and then create the future. They demand that each of us be our best and they include play, that universal spice, that is irresistible.

Dr. John Bagshaw, Covert Bailey, Thompson Barton, Dr. Dean Bellavia, Dr. Jeff Bland, Dr. Michael Colgan, Wayne Dyer, Randy Elliott, Sonny Elliott, Dr. George Eversaul, Dr. Larry Funt, Tim Gallwey, Joan Garbo, Dr. George Goodheart, Dr. Duane Grummons, Avrom King, Mike Kroske, Jack LaLanne, Richard Mackley, Rick Mercer, Bill Pearl, Dan Poynter, Dr. Tom Pitts, Michael Quas, Tony Robbins, Dr. Bob Rothan, Dr. Janet Travell, Dr. Ralph Weiss, Bob Young.

For their participation in the early reasearch: Dr. Tom Foster, Dr. Tom Muller, and the St. Charles Medical Center, Dr. Fred Boyle and the Central Oregon Community College.

Those people who continue to research for better, and more accurate methods to measure body composition.

My personal support team, for their patience, caring, energy and willingness to take care of others: Marla Jo Rasmussen, Jason Hardy, Cyndi Davis and Dixie Wagaman.

Pete O'brien, the cartoonist who created the characters. Robert Howard for his cover design, and Cathy Peters for her editing.

Becky Quas, who has matched my passion and commitment for this project; the partner we all need.

Juliana, who shares my life and our vision, is an inspiration and oustanding example of how well the concepts work.

Table of Contents

List of Figures

The Lean Body Promise is dedicated to the challenge
that each individual holds the key to the future
of mankind, and mankind holds the key
to the future, and the survival
of life on this planet.

Introduction

For years, people have read books and followed programs to find solutions for their problems with appearance, health and performance. Many of us can "get in shape", "lower cholesterol", have a "special diet plan" and we are still searching for a "miracle cure" that will give us lasting results. Confused and discouraged by false claims of the rapid improvement programs, and lost in terms of what direction to take, we struggle with the mystery of, "How to improve," when weight and shape changes never seem to last, or,"What should we do," when these changes just don't happen in the first place?

When lost in any area, we need an accurate map to determine where we are and which direction to take. We also need a method and tools, to get to our destination, and a compass to stay on course. With physical change as the destination, this book is your map, food and activity are your tools, and Lean Body Mass is your compass and guidance system.

The Lean Body Mass (LBM) is a special part of your body, that is not fat. Your Lean Body Mass has the power to get rid of fat, change your shape, improve performance and create energy.

The Lean Body Promise is arranged as a map to create a new awareness of your body, and a direction for your success. The first four chapters are filled with charts, maps, and the Lean Body Mass orientation system that will become the foundation for all you will accomplish.

Chapters Five and Six are the transition chapters that address challenges and setbacks before they happen, and help you plan for the action part of your program.

Chapter Seven and Eight are the keys to your future. Chapter Seven takes you from the grocery store to the kitchen table, with all choices based on your food preferences and goals. Chapter Eight creates the support systems and structure to guarantee success.

The Lean Body Promise, uses your own body to determine the best approach and steps to guide you to rapid and effective improvement. The steps from your "LBM to the right foods", provide consistent results because they are designed to let the body do what it always does: respond and move toward optimum performance in every situation. In other words, right now your body is operating at 100% peak efficiency, with your present food and activity.

For some of you, this means no restrictions, great energy, and top performance from your body. For others, it means carrying an extra 40 to 100 pounds of fat, and the body responds heroically, but is left exhausted day, after day.

The Lean Body Promise, allows you to be totally aware, responsible, and in charge of your own rate of change. There is no one else to blame or praise. It also allows you to balance the basics of any food program to your body, in a way that fits whatever activity or lifestyle you choose. There is an unconditional guarantee that comes with being human; and it states that the more you commit to improving, the more obstacles there will be to your progress.

Working with Lean Body Mass and food, in a new way, will eliminate many of the plateaus you have previously encountered. From time to time, your motivation will slow, a block will look insurmountable, and unforeseen circumstances will appear in your life to test your commitment. When this happens, and it will happen, you will be able to work through these situations during your improvement program, and use these blocks as tools to make future progress.

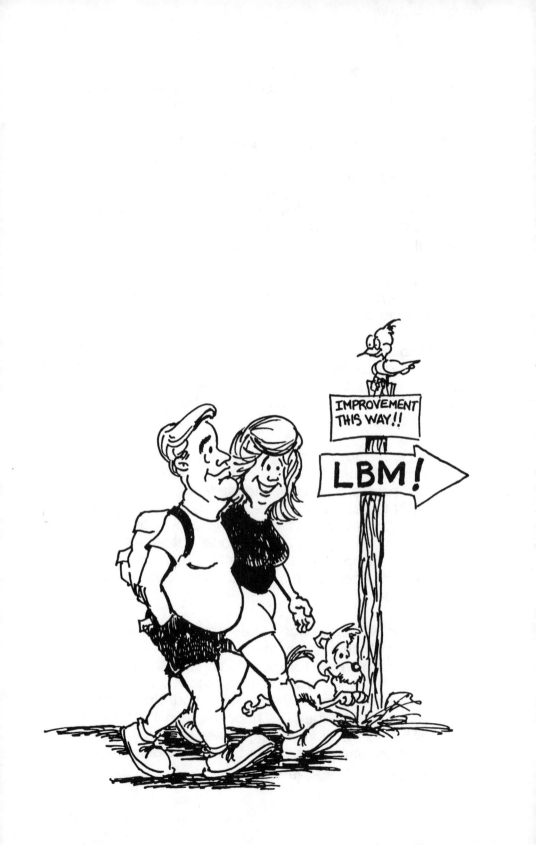

CHAPTER ONE

An Introduction to Your Body

*"Your Lean Body Mass **is** you; your fat is **on** you!"*

Overview

You are about to become involved in the most exciting and effective approach possible for improving your body. It works because the design is based on what other plans overlook--you as a unique individual. The solution to your weight and shape problems includes your activity level, your food choices and the most important part of your body: your Lean Body Mass.

When used properly, the information about your Lean Body Mass will be the foundation for all the steps in your improvement process. This process begins in Chapter One, and includes new and positive ways to look at your body and your true ideal weight. It also will establish what happens to your body when you are inactive and use incorrect eating programs, and how you can establish weight and shape goals that are realistic for you.

Body Compostion: What We're Made Of

Looking at bodies may be, if the truth were known, the greatest national and international pastime. Because attention to our own body and to other bodies already occupies so much of our time and is the basis for so many of our decisions, perhaps we can use this behavior in a new and useful way.

Visually, we perceive ourselves and others as slender, heavy, or perhaps muscular . . . in other words, a shape we like or a shape we do not like. Having a great or not-so-great shape is due to a difference between the amount and distribution of the two major parts of our body which determine shape: muscle and fat. Even though there are some skeletal differences in height and width, the main difference in shape and weight depends on the amount and arrangement of muscle and the amount and storage pattern of fat. The term "body com-position" refers to what the body is made of. The body composition evaluation is a method people use to deter-mine how much Lean Body Mass and how much fat they have in their bodies.

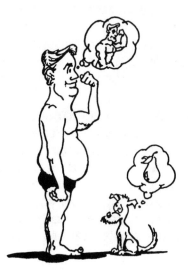

Researchers could suggest an infinite number of categories to describe various parts of the body. I suggest we divide the body into just two parts: the part we like and the part we don't like. The part of our body we like, enhances our appearance and shape, gives us energy, and provides us with the ability to heal and repair ourselves after injury. It also solves problems, handles stress, eats, enjoys relationships and life, touches and relates to the world. In other words, it is the part of our body that performs.

The part and the characteristics of our body we don't like are those that take away from our appearance, performance, shape and energy and prevent us from expressing our optimum potential.

What if we could identify, and even measure, the part of our body that we like? If we could learn more about this part, perhaps we could develop ways of using it for our own improvement. Also, if we could learn more about the part we don't like, we might be able to reduce, eliminate or de-emphasize this portion.

Fortunately, there is a way to identify and measure the part of our body we like. This portion, called the *Lean Body Mass*, can be described as follows: It is the part which needs food and activity, requires oxygen, moves around, thinks, feels and repairs itself. The rest of our body is, simply, fat. Fat does not need food, does not require oxygen, cannot generate activity, cannot repair itself, and, basically, is not alive. We might even say that your Lean Body Mass *is* you and the fat is *on* you.

Let's focus on the part of our body that is alive and has the ability to perform and function in the world. How much Lean Body Mass we have determines a great deal about how we look, feel and perform, as well as our level of energy and how rapidly changes can be made in weight, shape and performance.

Our bodies are composed of Lean Body Mass and fat. The Lean Body Mass is made of organs such as; skin, bone, liver, kidneys, heart and muscle. These organs change very little, during our adult years when we are in a normal state of health. When a change does occur in the Lean Body Mass, it can always be traced to an increase or decrease of muscle tissue. This is why I have chosen to emphasize the muscle portion of the Lean Body Mass as a measuring system for the body.

Another characteristic of muscle is that it never lies. It responds exactly to how it is nourished and used. Muscle might be compared to a relationship which will last if we spend time and take care of it. If we ignore or abuse the relationship, it slowly but certainly goes away.

The Importance of Muscle

If you want a stimulating conversation, apart from politics and religion, then bring up the subject of muscle. The word muscle itself can be intimidating in a way that is different from the word fat. We understand fat, or think we do, because it is what most of our weight/shape information and conversation is based upon. We don't understand muscle; yet, there is an uneasy feeling that we should know more. While at first we might not understand its value, we know at some level, muscle is very important.

Let's discuss muscle from a new perspective. The invitation here is to consider looking at muscle mass from an entirely new direction. This is much like an invitation to try a new thought (like a new flavor of ice cream). To do that, you have to set aside your old favorite thought (favorite flavor) for a moment. You can always have your old thought or flavor back; and you just might like the new one better.

When there is an increase or decrease of an adult's Lean Body Mass, it is a change in the muscle mass, not a change in the organs or bones. Muscle tissue makes up approximately 30-35% of the Lean Body Mass of the average adult female and approximately 40%-45% of the Lean Body Mass of the average adult male. Knowing how the muscle changes in response to our activity and diet programs is a key for those of us who want to stop searching and actually begin improving our bodies.

Muscle adapts to what we do. It could be thought of as a digital display or computer printout of what is happening to us on the inside. Under some negative conditions, muscle degenerates or goes away; during positive conditions, it develops or grows. (These conditions will be discussed later in the book.) Generally, a loss of Lean Body Mass is muscle. Knowing how much we have to start with can help us determine whether the body is degenerating, growing or maintaining.

The critical question to ask is, "How far into a state of deterioration does a person go before finding out and correcting the problem?" In a state of health, the muscle tissue of the body maintains or grows, adapting itself to its environment. Muscle responds to activity, to inactivity, and to the amount of food a person eats. This dynamic and changeable tissue reflects what the person has been doing to arrive at his or her present condition.

Muscle: Some Revealing Facts

I have chosen to define muscle by its function, rather than by its scientific names and chemical reactions. Do these definitions and descriptions fit your feeling of what muscle tissue is or could be?

- Muscle is a living tissue which uses a large amount of oxygen. This means that it is capable of using a large amount of calories under the right conditions.

- Muscle is an adaptive and changeable tissue. Example: Notice that a broken arm or leg appears smaller when the cast is removed, and then returns to its normal size after one or two months of normal activity.

- Muscle is the engine that powers our body's movements and determines our performance.

- Muscle will decrease if we are not eating or training correctly.

- Muscle becomes a convenient and available source of protein when we are not eating enough protein. Therefore, muscle will actually be broken down and used to provide protein for the rest of the body.

- Muscle becomes an available source of carbohydrates when we are not eating enough carbohydrates.

- Muscle is our body's furnace, which uses fat and carbohydrate for fuel.

- Muscle used during exercise at a correct Training Heart Rate (THR) will use fat as fuel.

- Muscle determines, and is in charge of, our performance and our shape.

- Muscle tone helps to eliminate aches and pains.

• Muscle helps the heart by acting as a pump, returning blood to the lungs for more oxygen. While arteries have elasticity and can force the blood on to its destination, the veins rely on muscle and physical activity to move the blood back to the heart.

• Our posture depends on muscle.

• Muscle **is** you; fat is **on** you.

• Under-muscled people are as great a health concern as over-fat people.

• Losing muscle is common, difficult to detect, and somewhat like dying slowly.

At some point we learn that our muscle is the result of what we do and how we eat. We then can choose to do something about our condition, or become satisfied with where we are.

Quality of Muscle Tissue

To demonstrate the presence of muscle and fat visually, I had a CAT scan X-ray taken through my legs and abdomen. A CAT scan is a cross section X-ray picture of parts of a person's body. (Figure 1, p. 22)

Like everyone else, my first interest was in how much fat was present, where it was, and how it looked on the film. The X-ray technician explained it was possible to determine the density of the various body tissues. It was apparent that the density of the fat on my stomach was less than the fat on my thighs. I have since learned that the fat on my thighs was more dense, or firm, because it had been present on my body much longer.

Figure 1 - CT Section, Adult Male 90% Lean Body Mass

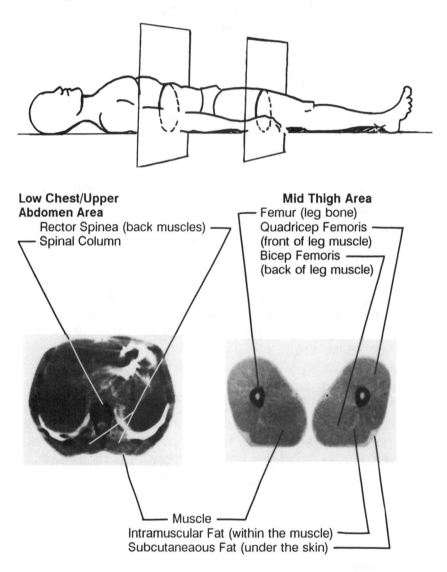

Low Chest/Upper Abdomen Area
Rector Spinea (back muscles)
Spinal Column

Mid Thigh Area
Femur (leg bone)
Quadricep Femoris (front of leg muscle)
Bicep Femoris (back of leg muscle)

Muscle
Intramuscular Fat (within the muscle)
Subcutaneaous Fat (under the skin)

Low Chest/Upper Abdomen Area: Notice the presence of back muscles next to the vertebrae. The fat underneath the skin is the lighter outside ring.

Mid Thigh Area: Notice the difference in the amount of muscle on the front of the leg compared to the amount on the back.

It was also clear that the muscle density was different on the front of my leg than it was on the back of my legs. Also, the leg muscle tissue was different from the muscle tissue surrounding the spinal column. (My spinal column muscles were less compact and weaker, because I avoided back exercises for many years.) After studying CAT scans of "average" adults, the following conditions were consistent: deterioration or absence of muscle; lack of muscle density; presence of fat, and increase of density in the fat tissue.

Figure 2 - CT Section, Adult Female, 50% Lean Body Mass

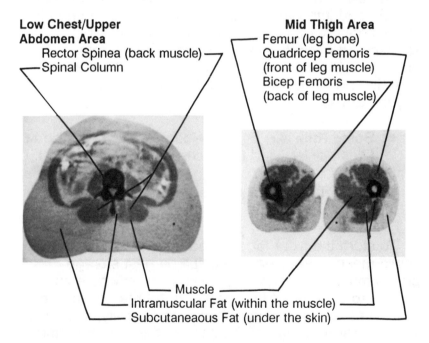

Low Chest/Upper Abdomen Area
Rector Spinea (back muscle)
Spinal Column

Mid Thigh Area
Femur (leg bone)
Quadricep Femoris (front of leg muscle)
Bicep Femoris (back of leg muscle)

Muscle
Intramuscular Fat (within the muscle)
Subcutaneaous Fat (under the skin)

Low Chest/Upper Abdomnen Area: Note the absence of muscle in the Spinal Erector Muscles and the light areas which are Intramuscular Fat. This person has had back problems for years.

Mid Thigh Area: Note the deterioration of the leg muscle, and the amount of Intramuscular and Surface Fat present. This is typical for a person with an inactive lifestyle.

Seeing muscle loss on the CAT scans created questions in my mind about the relationship of muscle to posture, to performance, and to chronic pain symptoms. What caused this muscle loss? What signs do we have that our muscles are deteriorating? What would prevent a decrease in Lean Body Mass? How can we replace the lost muscle once it is detected?

Body Fat: Two Basic Rules

Let's now turn our attention from muscle and Lean Body Mass to fat. The explanations for fat range from wordy scientific statements about genetic makeup, hormones, and intricate metabolic formulas to down-home statements like, "Everybody in my family has a big stomach!" It might be helpful to erase all previous opinions and beliefs about why our bodies look the way they do and adopt two new basic rules that can lead anyone to vast improvement.

- **Basic Rule #1:** Eat more calories than your body uses per day and the excess is deposited as fat.

- **Basic Rule #2:** The inactive part of the body stores the fat!

To store the extra fat, the body looks for a place that would make a great storage unit. The best storage places must have certain qualities. Look at where we choose to store our extra "stuff" around the house. We pick areas that have very little use and activity, such as a kitchen drawer, a part of the garage, the attic or certain closets.

When it comes to fat storage, the body looks for similar places. Please notice that fat is not deposited in our hands, forearms, feet or jaw muscles. If we lived in a society where we did not use our hands and feet, never spoke or chewed, and communicated, or moved around, by using our thighs, hips and waists, the result would be exactly the opposite of what we have now. We would have trim little waists, hips and thighs, with fat deposits in our hands, forearms, feet and jaws.

In this make-believe situation, the complaint would be, "Why can't I get rid of my fat forearms or chubby fingers?" Or, "Everybody in my family looks this way." At that point, researchers would develop theories, devise physiological equations and study hormones to decide why some people deposit more fat in their feet than in their forearms, and why males deposit their fat more in one area, and females more in another area.

Imagine what it would be like to visit earth from another planet, and look objectively at humans. We would watch people eat more than they could use in a day, under-exercise, and then complain about the result of excess fat on their bodies. As space visitors, we would write notes like these in our journals:

"Interesting life forms! They cause the problem and then complain because the problem exists. Then they use programs which are not effective and, therefore, lead to more complaints!"

A Deeper Look At Fat

Let's look at our body's fat from a new viewpoint. Fat is an extremely specialized fuel. This fuel can be consumed efficiently by a specific tissue, under certain conditions. The conditions are: physical activities called training, and the specific tissue is muscle. Any decrease in physical activity results in a decrease in muscle and an increase in body fat. To help our understanding, let's examine at where the fat is located on our bodies and why it is there.

Types of Body Fat

1. Essential fat: Unnoticeable

Essential fat is necessary for hormone production and other tasks. Do not worry about not having enough essential fat. The thinnest persons and even starvation victims, have essential fat.

> Where: Inside the cells and within the body where you cannot see it.

> How much: Three to 20 pounds, depending upon your age, size and sex.

2. Excess fat: Noticeable

It is the fat that is obvious and that we complain about.

> Where: Under the skin, called subcutaneous fat.

> How much: The amount is variable, from a few pounds to several hundred. Even small amounts are not popular with most people.

3. Excess fat: Hidden

Hidden fat is difficult to detect visually, and it accompanies a decrease in lean mass. The associated characteristics are; a decrease in performance and energy, excessive fatigue and the ability to gain weight easily.

> Where: Between muscle fibers called intramuscular fat. Hidden fat also appears next to the organs in the body cavity.

> How much: Again, variable amounts. This is the type of fat that thin people think they don't have.

Figure 3 - CT Section, Adult Male, 65% Lean Body Mass

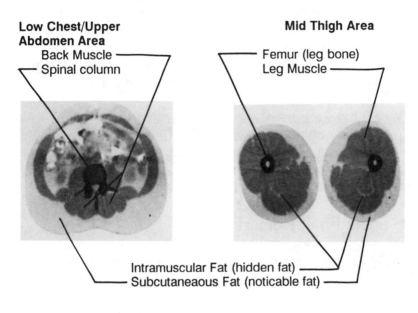

Why do we have excess fat?

One theory is that the body is busy stocking up for all the activity that is going to be done in the future, for the long, hard winter or for the upcoming famine. Unfortunately, and contrary to popular belief, human beings do not use stored fat for fuel when they stop eating.

There are definite drawbacks to a large amount of excess fat. Excess fat is:

● Not used as a food source by the body, most of the time.

● Perceived as unattractive.

● A block to optimum performance, because it is hard to function optimally when we carry nonvital tissue with us.

Other reasons people have excess fat relate to illness and inactivity. Regardless of how healthy we generally are, from time to time we can become ill. When we are ill, we can easily lose more muscle than fat. Only by monitoring our body composition, can we measuring what long-term effect illness has on our Lean Body Mass.

When the amount of muscle is reduced we cannot burn as many calories. If we cannot use all the calories in the food we eat, the excess is stored as fat. When we lose some muscle tissue, or do not use the muscle we have, we cannot use any of our extra body fat.

Fat: Some Final Remarks

Using our excess fat as fuel was part of the human's design developed thousands of years ago, seemingly by a group of engineers who did not conceive of our modern, inactive lifestyle. As technology advanced, people became less active and, therefore, needed less muscle. These engineers also did not foresee the convenience of prepackaged, concentrated and processed foods, which means we can eat more calories in less bites and less time.

Foods also are much more available these days. We have to forage only as far as the cupboard or refrigerator, compared with our ancestors foraging for days, to obtain a meal. If our activity level and calorie intake do not match our Lean Body Mass, an increase in body fat and/or a decrease in lean mass, (muscle) are unavoidable.

Fat, as a body tissue, is dormant and passive, and contributes nothing to a person's performance or aliveness. Traditional methods of weight and shape control focus on fat, see it as the enemy, and seek to remove the enemy by eliminating anything associated with it. In other words, food becomes Public Enemy #1.

I suggest that we focus our attention on the Lean Body Mass, specifically the muscle tissue. This is the alive part of our body. It uses oxygen and fuel (calories). It is the dynamic part that allows us to move, live, function and contribute. Learning to care for, nurture, and develop the muscle will be our best strategy for handling any problems we may encounter with fat.

Body Composition Evaluations

How much lean and fat mass we have determines how our body performs. The performance level and appearance of the body depend upon how it is fed and used. The effects of food and activity are clearly identified by a body composition evaluation. The evaluation can solve the mystery of whether or not a program is working.

People's resistance to body compostion evaluations shows up in the following ways:

> Most people do not want to be told "how fat" they are.
> They know . . . and would rather not discuss it.

First, people can be told how lean they are, not how fat they are. Everyone has lean mass. This is the exciting and alive part. Knowing how much lean mass you have is positive and motivating, and lets you develop a winning strategy for improving your body.

> People don't want to be told that what they are doing
> is wrong and that they will have to change.

Second, the results from a body composition evaluation help people improve their shape and weight. People can learn about food and training programs, and then choose a program according to what they like, and the information provided by a body compostition evaluation. Personal choice is the key to any decision-making process and the key to success.

The entire idea of testing is negative in our culture. Who wants to get a bad grade, even on a body composition evaluation?

Lastly, a body composition evaluation is not like other tests that emphasize what is wrong. It is designed to emphasize the Lean Body Mass, and the evaluation can be used for lifelong improvements!

Learning how much lean and fat we now have is the only way to know if there is a change next time we determine our body composition. When we lose muscle our energy and performance drop. A decrease in muscle tissue cannot be seen, and it is slow, so we don't feel it. A balance of food and activity to each individual's body will replace the muscle loss, or keep it from happening.

Research has proven one conclusive fact: being sedentary or inactive, under or overeating, illness, and under or overtraining guarantees a undesireable change. The change is inside where we cannot see it. The muscle mass can decrease as the fat increases, while the scale weight stays the same. The way to prevent fooling ourselves is to get a body composition evaluation.

Body Composition Methods

There are several methods of determining body composition. Certain methods take the entire body into account, while others take sample measurements at different body sites and use calculations to determine the whole body's composition.

Whole Body Measurements:

The original whole body method is hydrostatic weighing or water weighing. This method begins with a person sitting in a type of tub with his or her head above the surface. Then, in order to be weighed, the person's head must be placed under the water for a few seconds while someone records the weight.

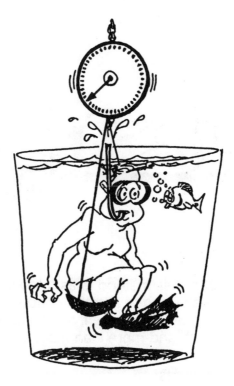

The concept of this method is as follows: The more Lean Body Mass one has, the heavier they are in water. Muscle is heavier and sinks in water, while fat is lighter and floats.

The second method of determining body composition is the impedance unit. A small sensor pad, connected to a monitor, is placed on the person's wrist and ankle. Then, an undetectable current is sent through the sensors. The fraction of a second required for the current to travel the length of the body gives that person's percent of lean and fat tissue on a computer print-out.

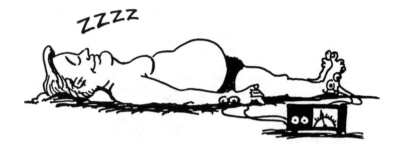

The concept of this method is as follows: Muscle contains more water and is a better conductor of electricity than fat. The current travels faster when there is less fat, and more lean mass present.

Spot Measurements:

Spot measurements are based on the amount of fat recorded at the various body sites.

The most commonly used method is the skin caliper. This is a device which gathers up and measures the thickness of fat and skin at specific spots on the body.

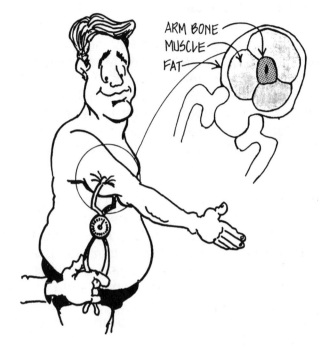

ARM BONE
MUSCLE
FAT

Another method is a sonar device which uses sound waves to determine the depth of fat between the muscle and skin.

A more recent technique uses light to penetrate through fat and muscle fibers, thus measuring their density and amount.

The concept of spot measurement methods is that the measurable surface fat or fat density at certain sites, reveals the amount of fat for the entire body.

Advantages and Disadvantages of Body Composition Methods

Hydrostatic Weighing: The advantage of the hydrostatic weighing system is accuracy. Most body composition standards are determined using the water tank. The disadvantage is that the technique of exhaling all air and lowering the head under the water for a few seconds is difficult to learn. Hydrostatic weighing also takes more time, and consistent results are influenced by the person's participation.

Impedance: An advantage of the impedance unit is that the person does not have to learn a technique for an accurate result. The method is less time-consuming and may be done with the person fully clothed. The disadvantage of this method is that varying amounts of water in the person's body affect the results. Instructions regarding how to get the most accurate results, using the impedance unit, are obtained from the person conducting the evaluation.

Skin Caliper: Advantages of the skin caliper method are: there is no required preparation and instruction, and eating or training before the evaluation does not affect the results. The disadvantage is that calipers measure surface fat at specific spots; thus the overall body composition is determined by a formula. Formulas will not provide an accurate result when there is excess fat in the muscle, when there is a loss of muscle, or when a person has an unusual fat storage pattern.

Sonar And Light Techniques: The disadvantages and advantages of these methods are similar to the skin calipers, because they are also a spot testing device. Consistent results for both methods depend on having the same spots measured at each evaluation.

Using Lean Mass to Improve

It is possible to become very attached to a particular body composition evaluation method and discount the other techniques. Any of the methods can an effective tool for your total program. The most accurate results can be obtained by keeping the following points in mind.

1. Be consistent and keep a daily journal of food and training.

2. Use the same body composition method each time.

3. Avoid a discussion of "which method is best." Instead, discuss what is working, in terms of your food and activity program and especially the results from your last three evaluations. This discussion provides useful information, creates possibilities for everyone and avoids the issue of right or wrong.

Consistency is the key issue in all body composition evaluations. It is important to maintain consistency in the method used and in the timing between evaluations. Evaluations can be done once a month, or at two week intervals to learn the results of food and training at a faster rate. The cost of an evaluation is slight compared with the money spent on club memberships and diet programs.

Figure Four (p. 36) is an example of a body composition report. Read the wording carefully. The report format will increase your awareness of Lean Body Mass concepts and establish a base for your future goals.

BODY COMPOSITION REPORT

Lean Body Mass (LBM) is the amount of muscle, organ and bone your body has. The LBM, which we measure in percentage or pounds, becomes the key number in your body composition. This number represents the vital and dynamic part of you. Why? Because it is the lean body mass that burns the calories, burns the fat, controls your weight, and controls your shape! Obviously your goal should be to have an ideal amount of lean mass for your body.

YOUR BODY COMPOSITION SCORES

Lean Body Mass _____%

Lean Body Mass _____lbs

Fat _____lbs

Total Scale Weight _____lbs

LEAN BODY MASS PERCENTAGES

	Inactive Range	Moderately Active Range	Athletic Range Optimum Performance
WOMEN	60% to 77%	75% to 84%	81% to 94%
MEN	75% to 84%	82% to 90%	87% to 95%

If you are not pleased with the body composition scores, you may consider reducing fat, increasing lean or both, depending upon your goals.

The LBM score is a very sensitive indicator of how well your training (exercise) or food programs are working.

You begin losing the muscle portion of your lean body mass with:

- Improper eating habits.
- Food restrictive plans (the popular diets).
- Over-training.
- Inactive or sedentary lifestyle.
- Illness.

A major consideration in your fitness goals should be to maintain or increase your LBM. This requires a program that you know is working. Your next Body Composition Evaluation will clearly determine is your food and exercise programs are moving you in the right direction.

The interval between body composition evaluations should be 2 - 4 weeks, depending on the rate of change you desire and the activity level you choose.

Figure 4 - Body Composition Report

Interpretation of the Report

While most body composition results are recorded in terms of a percentage of body fat, I prefer using the amount of Lean Body Mass. The report provides a starting point from which to measure future progress. We can use our individual bodies to develop a strategy for improvement based upon our own Lean Body Mass.

How do we know where to begin? Having an accurate starting point for an improvement strategy is absolutely critical. Have you ever been in the middle of a large shopping mall, completely disoriented about where you are? Soon you spot a small display, and inside there is a red arrow pointing to one section of the mall, with a sign saying, "You are Here." A body composition report also says "You are Here." It is an objective statement of where you are now--your starting point.

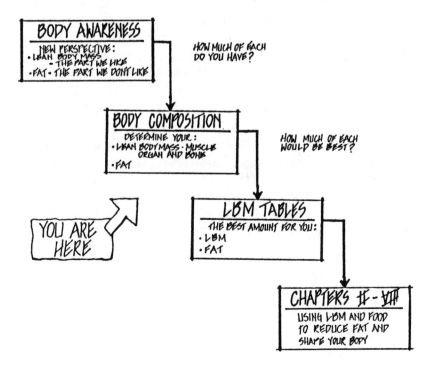

Body composition evaluations can be used to plan an effective strategy for improvement. The strategy allows food and activity to shape our bodies and control our weight. How much activity and how much food for each individual can only be planned using their Lean Body Mass. Not using the Lean Body Mass to plan improvement, can only be guesswork.

Body Composition: Some Final Thoughts

Age is not a limiting factor when we want to improve our body composition. The length of time we have been inactive has more influence on our Lean Body Mass than how old we are. Lean mass responds to our individual programs, regardless of age. You can develop an image for your body, and plan a strategy to accomplish your goals using your own Lean Body Mass.

What is the best percent of lean mass and fat? People consistently feel and perform better when men begin to approach body composition ranges of 90% lean mass or above, and women approach 83% lean mass or greater. Our bodies deserve the chance to express who we are, which cannot be done when performance is impaired by having too little muscle and too much fat.

For anyone who might not like their body after altering it, there is a "double-your-fat-back" guarantee built into the system. If you don't like how you look and feel at a higher percentage of Lean Body Mass, you can have your old body weight, shape and energy level back in just a few short months. You are in complete control!

The Height/Weight Tables

The standard height/weight tables state that for a certain frame size and height people should be a specific weight. (Figure 5, p. 40) These tables took the average height and weight of large groups of people to determine standard values. The weights of most people have been compared to this broad cross-section in the past. These tables have, at times, changed for various reasons. One example within the last ten years, is when an insurance company allowed a ten pound increase in each category simply because people could not maintain the weight standards set years ago.

Many organizations, institutions and health care providers determine employment and insurability according to these tables. Most diet plans determine calorie intake each day, using the height/weight tables. Even bathroom scales are purchased to compare weight to these tables. As with many of our standards, and because they have been the standard for so long, we have stopped looking for better ways to measure our weight.

We have always known there are vast differences in the weight and shape of our bodies; yet the standard height/weight tables lump everyone together and do not allow for our individuality. To control weight or shape, knowing your present amount of lean mass is the first step. Then you can use it to plan an individualized and accurate approach to improved body shape and weight.

The next question is, "What percentage of Lean Body Mass and fat should I be?" Your correct percentage is decided upon by you. Be realistic and allow time. An increase in lean mass, or decrease in fat, can only be accomplished by adhering to a food and activity plan designed according to your Lean Body Mass.

WOMEN Weight in Pounds (in indoor clothing; for nude weight deduct 2-4 lbs.)

Height (with shoes) Feet	Inches	Small Frame	Medium Frame	Large Frame
4	10	92- 98	96-107	104-119
4	11	94-101	98-110	106-122
5	0	96-104	101-113	109-125
5	1	99-107	104-116	112-128
5	2	102-110	107-119	115-131
5	3	105-113	110-122	118-134
5	4	108-116	113-126	121-138
5	5	111-119	116-130	125-142
5	6	114-123	120-135	129-146
5	7	118-127	124-139	133-150
5	8	122-131	128-143	137-154
5	9	126-135	132-147	141-158
5	10	130-140	136-151	145-163
5	11	134-144	140-155	149-168
6	0	138-148	144-159	153-173

STANDARD HEIGHT WEIGHT TABLE
BASED ON SCALE WEIGHT

MEN Weight in Pounds (in indoor clothing; for nude weight deduct 5-7 lbs.)

Height (with shoes) Feet	Inches	Small Frame	Medium Frame	Large Frame
5	2	112-120	118-129	126-141
5	3	115-123	121-133	129-144
5	4	118-126	124-136	132-148
5	5	121-129	127-139	135-152
5	6	124-133	130-143	138-156
5	7	128-137	134-147	142-161
5	8	132-141	136-152	147-166
5	9	136-145	142-156	151-170
5	10	140-150	146-160	155-174
5	11	144-154	150-165	159-179
6	0	148-158	154-170	164-184
6	1	152-162	158-175	168-189
6	2	156-167	162-180	173-194
6	3	160-171	167-185	178-199
6	4	164-175	172-190	182-204

STANDARD HEIGHT WEIGHT TABLE
BASED ON SCALE WEIGHT

Figure 5 - Height/Weight Tables for Women and Men

The Lean Body Mass Tables

The Lean Body Mass table lets us determine weight according to our individual bodies and our activity levels. The table also serves as a checkpoint to measure our progress, and establish if our current program is working.

How to Determine Your Optimum Weight:

The Lean Body Mass tables will allow you to calculate your weight using your present lean mass. (Figures 6-7, p. 42-43) You will also see that by changing the activity level, lean mass or fat, you can consider multiple options for lean mass and fat amounts. This will be an exercise in looking at the possibilities for your future body.

1. Start with your present lean mass. Decide if there are some changes you would like to make in your weight or shape. For example, we will assume you are 135 pounds, 5' 3" and have 85 pounds of Lean Body Mass. We further assume that you would like to decrease your weight and improve your shape by reducing the amount of fat on your hips and thighs.

2. Consider two possibilities:

(a) Maintain your present lean mass and reduce your fat to a lower percentage. (Check Lean Body Mass table for men and women.) Is this a good weight for you? Is this too light? If this weight is too light . . . then consider "b" below.

(b) Select the weight you would like to be. Check the appropriate lean mass, according to your activity level. If your present lean mass is too low, your goal would be to increase lean. For example, you are now 135 pounds in the moderately active range and would like your scale weight to be 120 pounds. If you look in the left-hand column at your desired weight of 120 pounds, and then to the lean mass column, you will find that 95 pounds of lean mass is necessary, which requires a gain of 10 pounds of muscle.

LEAN BODY MASS TABLE FOR WOMEN

ACTIVITY LEVEL

Scale Weight lbs	Inactive Range (60% to 77%) Lean Mass lbs		Moderately Active Range (75% to 84%) Lean Mass lbs		Athletic Range Optimum Performance (81% to 94%) Lean Mass lbs	
90	54.0	69.3	67.5	75.6	72.9	84.6
95	57.0	73.1	71.2	79.8	76.9	89.3
100	60.0	77.0	75.0	84.0	81.0	94.0
105	63.0	80.8	78.7	88.2	85.0	98.7
110	66.0	84.7	82.5	92.4	89.1	103.4
115	69.0	88.5	86.2	96.6	93.1	108.1
120	72.0	92.4	90.0	100.8	97.2	112.8
125	75.0	96.2	93.7	105.0	101.2	117.5
130	78.0	100.1	96.5	109.2	105.3	122.2
135	81.0	103.9	101.2	113.4	109.3	126.9
140	84.0	107.8	105.0	117.6	113.4	131.3
145	87.0	111.7	108.7	121.8	117.4	136.3
150	90.0	115.5	112.5	126.0	121.5	141.0
155	93.0	119.4	116.2	130.2	125.5	145.7
160	96.0	123.2	120.0	134.4	129.6	150.4
165	99.0	127.1	123.7	138.6	133.6	155.1
170	102.0	130.9	127.5	142.8	137.7	159.8
175	105.0	134.8	131.2	147.0	141.7	164.5
180	108.0	138.6	135.0	151.2	145.8	169.2
190	114.0	146.3	142.5	159.6	153.9	178.6
200	120.0	154.0	150.0	168.0	162.0	188.0
210	126.0	161.7	157.5	176.4	170.1	197.4
220	132.0	169.4	165.0	184.8	178.2	206.8
230	138.0	177.1	172.5	193.2	186.3	216.2
240	144.0	184.8	180.0	201.6	194.4	225.6
250	150.0	192.5	187.5	210.0	202.5	235.0

To Find: **YOUR IDEAL WEIGHT — WITH YOUR PRESENT LEAN BODY MASS.**
• Select your activity level.
• Move down the column to your current LBM.
• Look to the far left under scale weight for your "ideal" weight.

To Find: **YOUR IDEAL LEAN BODY MASS**
• Locate your present or fantasy weight in the "scale weight " column.
• Move across to the correct activity level.
• This number is the LBM necessary for your best shape and weight and energy —at this activity level.

("Ideal" varies with personal choice.)

Figure 6 - Lean Body Mass Table for Women

LEAN BODY MASS TABLE FOR MEN

ACTIVITY LEVEL

Scale Weight lbs	Inactive Range (75% to 84%) Lean Mass lbs		Moderately Active Range (82% to 90%) Lean Mass lbs		Athletic Range Optimum Performance (87% to 95%) Lean Mass lbs	
130	97.5	109.2	107.6	117.0	113.1	123.5
135	101.2	113.4	110.7	121.5	117.4	128.2
140	105.0	117.6	114.8	126.0	121.8	133.0
145	108.7	121.8	118.9	130.5	126.1	137.7
150	112.5	126.0	123.0	135.0	130.5	142.5
155	116.2	130.2	127.1	139.5	134.8	147.2
160	120.0	134.4	131.2	144.0	139.2	152.0
165	123.7	138.6	135.3	148.5	143.5	156.7
170	127.5	142.8	139.4	153.0	147.9	161.5
175	131.2	147.0	143.5	157.5	152.2	166.2
180	135.0	151.2	147.6	162.0	156.6	171.0
185	138.7	155.4	151.7	166.5	160.9	175.7
190	142.5	159.6	155.8	171.0	165.3	180.5
195	146.2	163.8	159.9	175.5	169.6	185.2
200	150.0	168.0	164.0	180.0	174.0	190.0
205	153.7	172.2	168.1	184.3	178.3	194.7
210	157.5	176.4	172.2	189.0	182.7	199.5
215	161.2	180.6	176.3	193.5	187.0	204.2
220	165.0	184.8	180.4	198.0	191.4	209.0
230	172.5	193.2	188.6	207.0	200.1	218.5
240	180.0	201.6	196.8	216.0	208.8	228.0
250	187.5	210.0	205.0	225.0	217.5	237.5
260	195.0	218.4	213.2	234.0	227.2	247.0
270	202.5	226.8	221.1	243.0	234.9	256.5
280	210.0	235.2	229.6	252.0	243.6	266.0
290	217.5	243.6	237.8	261.0	252.3	275.5
300	225.0	252.0	246.0	270.0	261.0	285.0

To Find: **YOUR IDEAL WEIGHT - WITH YOUR PRESENT LEAN BODY MASS.**
• Select your activity level.
• Move down the column to your current LBM.
• Look to the far left under scale weight for your "ideal" weight.

To Find: **YOUR IDEAL LEAN BODY MASS**
• Locate your present or fantasy weight in the "scale weight " column.
• Move across to the correct activity level.
• This number is the LBM necessary for your best shape and weight and energy —at this activity level.

("Ideal" varies with personal choice.)

Figure 7 - Lean Body Mass Table for Men

Example Comparisons

The following sections allows you to visualize the concepts already presented in Chapter One. The example's are paired to demonstrate the incompleteness of scale weight and the recommendation of the standard Height/Weight Tables. For Example, the daily calories based on the tables do not distinguish between fat weight and lean weight.

Compare the values for height, weight and Lean Body Mass and observe the difference in appearance. Look beyond the obvious differences in size and observe shape and fat distribution patterns.

Observe how one person may weigh considerably less and yet be "fatter" (Figure 8, p. 45). Daily calories used based on weight alone is misleading.

Notice that persons with the same height and body composition percentage look different due to the actual amount of lean and fat pounds (Figure 9, p. 46). Where is the fat on the "thin" person? Calorie requirements in this case are influenced by Lean Body Mass differences.

Persons with the same amount of Lean Body Mass and similar heights may vary dramatically due to the quantity of fat present (Figure 10, p. 47).

Confusion surrounding goal setting for ideal weight and having a direction to follow is made clear by an accurate analysis of body composition in addition to scale weight. An understanding of what we are made of and what we have to work with completes the picture and gives us confidence to achieve our goals.The standard Height/Weight tables and Lean Body Mass Tables make dramatically different calorie recommendations. What is the realistic outcome of these recommendations? How would you coach these people to achieve their goals?

FIGURE 8:

Both women are similar in height and 25 lbs. different in weight. The difference in weight is the amount of Lean Body Mass. Compare each person's goals and calories per day according to Lean Body Mass and Height/Weight tables.

Example A	**Example B**
HEIGHT • 5'0"	HEIGHT • 5'2"
WEIGHT 125#	WEIGHT 100#

STANDARD HEIGHT / WEIGHT TABLE

According to this table:
Example A should weigh 100#
Example B should weigh 106#

LEAN BODY MASS TABLE

According to this table using 80% LBM & 20% fat and their current LBM in pounds:
Example A should weigh 125#
Example B should weigh 87.5#

CALORIES USED PER DAY
Rest + Light Work + 1 Hr. Training

Based on Height/Weight Table:
Example A uses 1972 calories/day
Example B uses 1653 calories/day

Based on LBM Tables:
Example A uses 1440 calories/day
Example B uses 1008 calories/day

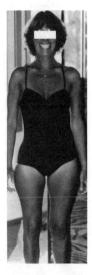

LEAN BODY MASS 100#	LEAN BODY MASS 70#
FAT - 25#	FAT - 30#
LBM % - 80%	LBM % - 70%

Example A's Goals are to appear slim and lose weight. In order to reach her ideal weight of of 100 lbs and maintain a 80% lean to 20% fat ratio, she would have to lose 20 lbs of LBM and 5 lbs of fat. This would severely decrease her energy level and her shape would remain the same. Another option is to maintain her present 100 lbs of LBM and reduce her fat 10-20 lbs. Not only would her strength and energy increase, she will also improve her shape and lose weight.

POINT: A weight of 105 lbs is not realistic with 100 lbs of Lean Body Mass.

Example B's Goals are to improve her shape and maintain her weight. Reaching her goal would require a 10 lb increase in LBM and a 10 lb decrease in body fat. This would give her an 80% lean 20% fat ratio and improve her shape and energy. Through monitoring her LBM, training and food, her weight gain would be muscle while decreasing her fat at the same time.

POINT: 70 lbs of LBM is inadequate to accomplish the desired goals.

Figure 8 - Example Comparison

FIGURE 9:

Both women are the same height, 5' 4". However, they are different in weight and shape. The thin woman appears underweight and the other appears average. The Height/Weight tables do not show the difference between muscle and fat. Therefore, it would be difficult to advise either woman how to achieve her goal. What would happen to the shape of their bodies if you took their fat away? As in Example 1, compare the calories and goals of each woman.

Example A
HEIGHT • 5'4"
WEIGHT 130#

Example B
HEIGHT • 5'4"
WEIGHT 83#

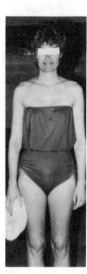

STANDARD HEIGHT / WEIGHT TABLE

According to this table:
Example A should weigh 120#
Example B should weigh 120#

LEAN BODY MASS TABLE

According to this table using 80% LBM & 20% fat and their current LBM in pounds:
Example A should weigh 130#
Example B should weigh 83#

CALORIES USED PER DAY
Rest + Light Work + 1 Hr. Training

Based on Height/Weight Table:
Example A uses 1972 calories/day
Example B uses 1653 calories/day

Based on LBM Tables:
Example A uses 1440 calories/day
Example B uses 1008 calories/day

LEAN BODY MASS 104#
FAT - 26#
LBM % - 80%

LEAN BODY MASS 66#
FAT - 17#
LBM % - 80%

Example A's Goal is to weigh 120 lbs and improve her shape. (1) At 120 lbs 80% lean, she would have to lose 8 lbs of lean mass and 2 lbs of fat which would not change her present shape. (2) At 120 lbs she could maintain her 104 lbs of LBM and focus on fat loss. This would improve her shape and she will achieve her complete goal.

Example B's Goal is to weigh 120 lbs and have a better shape. (1) This means a 37 lb increase in fat or a 30 lb increase in lean mass and a 7 lb increase in fat. Random weight gain without proper training will result in an excess fat gain and an undesirable shape. (2) At 120 lbs this woman could also increase her lean mass 37 lbs and keep her fat at 17 lbs, which would give her more muscle definition.

POINT: LBM provides greater accuracy and direction for the improvement of both women.

Figure 9 - Example Comparison

FIGURE 10:

Both women have the same Lean Body Mass and a 50 pound difference in weight. The difference in shape between this mother and daughter is due to the amount of body fat. Compare their calories determined by the Height/Weight and their Lean Body Mass tables.

<table>
<tr><td align="center">Example A
HEIGHT • 5'4"
WEIGHT 155#</td><td align="center">Example B
HEIGHT • 5'2"
WEIGHT 105#</td></tr>
</table>

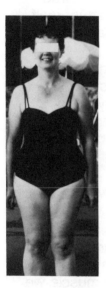

STANDARD HEIGHT / WEIGHT TABLE

According to this table:
Example A should weigh 120#
Example B should weigh 113#

LEAN BODY MASS TABLE

According to this table using 80% LBM &
20% fat and their current LBM in pounds:
Example A should weigh 112.5#
Example B should weigh 112.5#

CALORIES USED PER DAY
Rest + Light Work + 1 Hr. Training

Based on Height/Weight Table:
Example A uses 2305 calories/day
Example B uses 1721 calories/day

Based on LBM Tables:
Example A used 1296 calories/day
Example B used 1296 calories/day

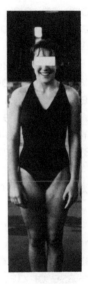

LEAN BODY MASS 90# FAT - 65# LBM % - 53%	LEAN BODY MASS 90# FAT - 15# LBM % - 88%

Example A's Goal is to weigh 120 lbs. This would require a 6 lb gain of lean body mass and a 41 lb loss of fat.

Example B is satisfied with her appearance and performance at 88% lean and 12% fat. For her to achieve the standard (20% fat and 80% lean), she would have to gain 6 lbs of fat and lose 6 lbs of muscle. Could she be convinced to add more fat to achieve a standard ideal?

POINT: Which table would you recomend using for a weight loss program?

POINT: The standard for percent of LBM and fat is really based on personal choice.

Figure 10 - Example Comparison

Goal and Achievement Chart

The next chart will become your reference page for future change. The information to be filled out is self-motivating. And, as a further source of motivation, I suggest you place a photograph of yourself now and a picture that represents your future body, over the instructions on this page. You will never again look at yourself as you are now without realizing your potential.

As you begin to determine your ideal weight and your ideal Lean Body Mass, a number of concerns may appear, and you may begin to doubt your ability to improve. Before becoming discouraged in advance or making decisions about what you "think" will not work, review the information on the next few pages.

Lean Body Mass: Your Guide for Positive Change

The performance and body we want depends upon the muscle portion of the Lean Body Mass, and not upon fat. Because changes in Lean Body Mass are an increase or decrease of muscle, the amount of muscle we have gained, lost or are losing is a major consideration in accomplishing our goals.

Our bodies change whether we want them to or not. That change is in constant harmony with our activity and what we eat. This makes our bodies, and what we do, a mirror for each other. Due to our modern lifestyle, occasional illness and frequent diets, the average adult has lost and continues to lose Lean Body Mass. Therefore, a body composition evaluation is one of the most meaningful reports we can get to inform us where we are, as a result of our lifestyles.

GOALS & ACHIEVEMENT CHART

		RATE OF IMPROVEMENT					
DATE:		**3 MOS.**	**6 MOS.**	**9 MOS.**	**12 MOS.**	**24 MOS.**	**36 MOS.**
BODY COMP REPORT:	**CURRENT**						
WEIGHT #	210						
LBM #	129						
FAT #	81						
MEASUREMENTS:							
NECK							
CHEST / BUST							
ARM — LEFT / RIGHT							
WAIST							
HIPS							
THIGH — LEFT / RIGHT							
CALF — LEFT / RIGHT							
OTHER							
TRAINING:							
AEROBIC — BIKE							
RUN							
SWIM							
DANCE							
OTHER							
RESISTANCE —							
FREE WEIGHTS							
MACHINES—							
UNIVERSAL/NAUTILIS							
OTHER							
PERFORMANCE GOALS:							

CURRENT BODY
(Photo)

FUTURE BODY
(Photo)

Figure 11 - Goal and Achievement Chart

Case Histories

Accurate Lean Body Mass information in the hands of a responsible person and a knowledgeable coach can result in consistent improvement. It also can answer many of the questions we have about ourselves such as:

- Why can't I lose weight?

- Why are my thighs so big?

- How can I lose my fat stomach?

- Why isn't this program working?

- How can my friend eat so much and not gain weight?

- Why am I always tired?

- Why can't I gain weight?

- The charts say I should weigh 25 pounds less than I do. Is this right?

Reviewing some case histories might illustrate how your participation and the body composition reports can create the change you want.

The Inactive Adult Male

This 36-year-old male is an excellent example of what happens to an alarming number of inactive adults. The executive's main complaint was:

"I cannot lose weight. I seem to be more tired lately, I have no energy and my pants keep shrinking in the waist."

At age 22 this man weighed 220 pounds (85% Lean Body Mass) and was a starting linebacker on his college football team. Eighty-five percent lean would be 187 pounds of Lean Body Mass and 33 pounds of fat.

At age 36 he weighed 200 pounds, 64% Lean Body Mass and 36% fat. His body composition was 128 pounds of Lean Body Mass and 72 pounds of fat. A 59 pound decrease in lean and a 39 pound increase in fat would certainly explain his lack of energy and his inability to lose weight.

His goal is to regain his former ratio of lean to fat (85% lean, and 15% fat), and maintain his present weight of 200 pounds. This would improve his appearance and increase his energy, strength and stamina. By comparing the two directions he could take his goal was clarified. He chose his program based on the type of changes he wanted for his body.

The Lean Body Mass approach helped to clarify another important point in this man's overall program. The standard calorie charts from the Height/Weight Tables list the daily calories for this size person at 3300 per day. His lean mass, which is the only part of the body capable of using calories, can use approximately 1800 per day. He thought that eating 2000 calories per day was undereating, and would help reduce his waist. In reality, according to his lean mass, he is overeating 200 calories each day and actually gaining weight.

The body composition evaluation allowed him to put his program into the proper framework for his own body. He could see that gaining lean mass was as important to his long term success as losing fat. He now has a way to measure the results of his food and exercise program.

His main goal is to be 85% lean, and 15% fat. There are two directions he could choose to reach his desired percentage:

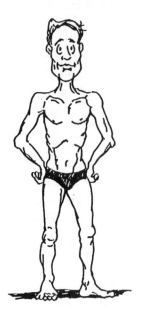 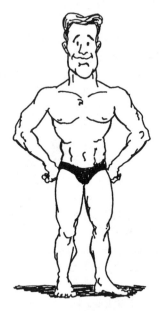

1. Maintain 128 pounds of Lean Body Mass (85%) and reduce his fat to 16 pounds (15%). His goal for weight is 200 pounds not 144 pounds. Therefore, 144 pounds would not work.

2. Increasing his Lean Mass to 170 pounds and reducing his amount of fat to 30 pounds would result in a body composition of 85% Lean Body Mass and a weight of 200.

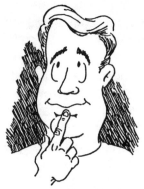

Figure 12 - Case History, the inactive adult male

Two Ways to be Fat

Both people on the following page have the same goals: they want attractive, energetic, appealing bodies. Both women are willing to make changes in their food and training program. What would you advise?

Both women have the same percentage of lean (50%) and fat (50%). The woman on the left has 98 pounds of lean mass to reduce fat and shape her body. The smaller woman on the right has 48 pounds of Lean to reduce her fat and improve her body.

Is one of these people in more trouble than the other from the standpoint of weight? Definitely YES, and it is not the larger of the two. The 195 pound person is much better off than the thin person. Remember, we are em-phasizing the part of you that is alive and uses calories, the lean mass. Therefore, if we focus on body fat and the person's appearance, it is possible to miss the amount of lean and provide inaccurate coaching. After all, haven't we been conditioned to think that thin is best?

The woman on the right has been dieting and under-eating for years. The result is a slender appearance. The loss of muscle has made it difficult for her to have the level of energy and performance she wants and anything she eats causes her to gain weight. It is challenging to overcome a mindset that states: The only way to stay small is to diet and undereat.

When there is a decrease in muscle mass the calories one consumes must change to balance with this loss. Any unused calories are stored in the body as fat. Only a planned food and training program with frequent body composition evaluations convinced this woman that eating more food and using training could change her from a skinny "fat" person to the energetic and shapely woman she wants to be.

FIGURE 12: Two Ways to Be Fat

There is a 2" difference in height and a 100 lb weight difference. Traditional standards say that the thin woman is normal and the other needs to lose weight. However, both women are the same percentage of lean mass and fat . As in the previous examples, compare the goals, current weight and calories both women use per day according to Lean Body Mass and the Height/Weight tables.

Example A
HEIGHT • 5'5"
WEIGHT 195#

Example B
HEIGHT • 5'3"
WEIGHT 95#

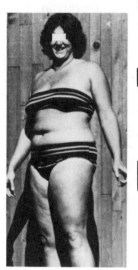

STANDARD HEIGHT / WEIGHT TABLE

According to this table:
Example A should weigh 121#
Example B should weigh 109#

LEAN BODY MASS TABLE

According to this table using 80% LBM &
20% fat and their current LBM in pounds:
Example A should weigh 122.5#
Example B should weigh 60#

CALORIES USED PER DAY
Rest + Light Work + 1 Hr. Training

Based on Height/Weight Table:
Example A uses 2672 calories/day
Example B uses 1609 calories/day

Based on LBM Tables:
Example A uses 1440 calories/day
Example B uses 720 calories/day

LEAN BODY MASS 98#
FAT - 97#
LBM % - 50%

LEAN BODY MASS 48#
FAT - 47#
LBM % - 50%

Example A's Goals are to lose weight and improve her shape. To achieve this goal she would needs to lose 73 lbs of body fat and maintain her lean mass. The lean mass gives the body its contours.

Example B's Goals are to improve her shape and increase energy. This person is already at her desired weight. A change from her present LBM to 80% LBM would mean a 28 lb increase of LBM and a 28 lbs decrease of fat.

POINT: Rather than place all emphasis and value on total scale weight or even percentage of LBM, a more important starting point is the pounds of Lean Body Mass!

Figure 13 - Case History, two ways to be fat

Your Personal Program: How to Start

You will benefit by having a coach to help you through the various stages of your program. Choosing this person is a most important step in your improvement package. Your coach may be an employee of a health club, your doctor or a competent friend.

Your coach has the following obligations:

1. To encourage accurate body composition evaluations to determine your starting point and monitor your progress.

2. To provide the most current and personalized information for your improvement.

3. To be the example! This should be your main criteria for selecting the person you will work with initially. Again, the coach must an example of health and of how well the information works.

You have the following obligations:

1. To recognize that your personal choice is the major factor. Will you move beyond average and explore the possibility of something more?

2. To be constantly aware that only your efforts in starting and continuing a correct food and training plan will allow continuous and permanent improvement.

3. To make a commitment to yourself. This depends upon your willingness to be responsible for your present condition, so you can be responsible for your success.

What's Possible for You?

You may already have the body you want and it is simply hiding, similar to the sculpture hidden inside a block of marble. Just as the sculpture requires a sculptor to reveal its presence, your Lean Body Mass is counting on you to recognize and reveal its presence. As a matter of fact, you are the only one who can do the work. Food and training are your tools; and, in this situation, you are both the sculptor and the marble.

Wrapping Up

Before reading this chapter, you probably had questions about your weight and shape that had never been answered, or even discussed. Learning about Lean Body Mass creates a new awareness of your body. An understanding of lean mass explains why muscle disappears when food and activity are not balanced. You also, by now, have the exciting sense of responsibility for the entire amount of muscle and fat on your body.

A body composition evaluation can establish a realistic goal for your weight. Follow-up body compositions create the opportunity for you to experiment with any food or training program, and always know the results by what happens to the most sensitive indicator of your progress--your Lean Body Mass.

People who monitor their body composition at least every four weeks will have accurate, up-to-date, information about their rate of change in body shape and weight. Chapter One is the compass that directs you out of the confusion that surrounds most weight/shape programs. The remaining chapters are designed to be guideposts, which encourage your participation, save you time, challenge your curiosity and involve you in the choices that create your future body.

CHAPTER 2

The Relationship Between Food And How You Look

"Our shape is not a random coincidence; it is a result!"

Overview

How the body is shaped and performs depends upon the muscle portion of the Lean Body Mass. Improving body shape depends on our activity level, combined with the quality and quantity of food we eat. I am emphasizing food at this point because we eat every day and we do not necessarily exercise every day. That which we do most often will have a greater influence on our weight and shape.

Our present Lean Body Mass determines the amount of calories (food energy) our bodies use each day. The calories used daily help us choose the amount of food we will eat each day to accomplish our goals. The point is that the most alive part of our body, the Lean Body Mass, tells us how much food to eat in an accurate, simple and straightforward way.

The Nature of Calories

Experts have contradicting opinions about how much food, how many calories, and how much of each particular food component--protein, fat and carbohydrates-- we should eat. In the ongoing confusion, it seems as though everyone has forgotten to consult with the most important expert of all . . . our Lean Body Mass.

If we are not consuming calories correctly, the Lean Body Mass will shrink and disappear. By using body composition and Lean Body Mass data, we can monitor the rate and direction of our progress.

How Much Food

The main concern for most of us is: "How many calories can we eat without gaining weight?" It would be important to address two other questions first. Just what are food calories and what is their purpose? A number of people explain calories as follows:

- "Calories mean fat on my body!"

- "Calories are what I avoid when I'm dieting."

- "Calories are in the food I'm not allowed to eat."

- "Calories make the wrong food taste good."

- "Calories are the bad guys."

Expressing an opinion about calories in a negative sense is common. Since calories are equated with food, eliminating calories means eliminating food. This negative concept of restriction and denial forms the basis for most diet and food plans. Let's take a new look at calories from the standpoint of Lean Body Mass.

- The muscle portion of the LBM is the engine and needs fuel in the form of food to function. The energy supplied by food is measured in calories.

- A certain amount of calories each day, and each meal are necessary. Too many calories can mean an increase in body fat and too few calories can mean a decrease in Lean Body Mass.

- Can you guess what the body uses for energy when you don't eat enough, or when you go on the latest diet? The body uses its own muscle. The body breaks down muscle to supply enough fuel for the brain and other tissues to function. The body actually takes muscle protein, converts it into carbohydrates, then uses it as very expensive brain and muscle fuel. Simply Stated:

"Either you eat enough calories to fuel your body or your body will take what it needs from your muscle."

So, calories really are the good guys. They are units of energy and we need them to survive, function and perform at our best. The next step is learning how many calories we need, based on our Lean Body Mass.

The Calorie Table, (Figure 14, p. 61) is based upon LBM, not total weight. We use LBM to determine the number of calories to eat, because total scale weight includes fat, which does not use calories. The number of calories the LBM uses will become the starting point for designing an optimum eating program.

The Calorie Table

The first step is to determine how many calories the body uses on a given day. The calories are calculated according to your amount of LBM and activities during a 24-hour period.

Explanation of the Calorie Table Headings:

Lean Body Mass in Pounds: Pounds of LBM

Base Calories per 24 Hours: The number of calories used by the Lean Body Mass every 24 hours. A day with very little activity results in the LBM using approximately this many calories just to fuel body processes.

Work 8-10 Hours: The next three columns are for the additional energy we expend during 8 to 10 hours of work. The amounts are added to our base calories.

Training per Hour: The next three columns are for training or exercise. Note how the calories used per hour relates to the Lean Body Mass.

Column 1: T.H.R. 50%-60%

The calories are based on aerobic activity at a 50% to 60% "Training Heart Rate" (T.H.R.). The lower T.H.R. will use a higher percentage of body fat.

Column 2: T.H.R. 65%-85%

The calories are based on aerobic activity at a 65% to 85% Training Heart Rate. At this pace, the average exerciser will use a higher percentage of carbohydrates. The accomplished distance athlete will use more fat at a higher T.H.R..

Column 3: WT.TR. 1 min.-rest

The calories in this column are for anaerobic activity, which is sometimes termed resistance or weight training. Weight training, with a one minute rest between exercises, uses carbohydrate for fuel and is not considered a fat loss activity. Increased fat loss does occur during the next 12 to 24 hours due to the muscle stimulation from training.

CALORIE TABLE

Based Upon Your Lean Body Mass — LBM

MASS IN POUNDS	BASE PER 24 HOURS	WORK 8 - 10 HOURS			TRAINING PER HOUR			CALORIES PER DAY
		LIGHT SITTING	CONSTANT WALKING	MANUAL LABOR	T.H.R. 50% - 60%	T.H.R. 65% - 85%	1 - min. REST	
50	600	120	180	300	180	240	210	
55	660	132	198	330	198	264	231	
60	720	144	216	360	216	288	252	
65	780	156	234	390	234	312	273	
70	840	168	252	420	252	336	294	
75	900	180	270	450	270	360	315	
80	960	192	288	480	288	384	336	
85	1020	204	306	510	306	408	357	
90	1080	216	324	540	324	432	378	
95	1140	228	342	570	342	456	399	
100	1200	240	360	600	360	480	420	
105	1260	252	378	630	378	504	441	
110	1320	264	396	660	396	528	462	
115	1380	276	414	690	414	552	483	
120	1440	288	432	720	432	576	504	
125	1500	300	450	750	450	600	525	
130	1560	312	468	780	468	624	546	
135	1620	324	486	810	486	648	567	
140	1680	336	504	840	504	672	588	
145	1740	348	522	870	522	696	609	
150	1800	360	540	900	540	720	630	
155	1860	372	558	930	558	744	651	
160	1920	384	576	960	576	768	672	
165	1980	396	594	990	594	792	693	
170	2040	408	612	1020	612	816	714	
175	2100	420	630	1050	630	840	735	
180	2160	432	648	1080	648	864	756	
185	2220	444	666	1110	666	888	777	
190	2280	456	684	1140	684	912	798	
195	2340	468	702	1170	702	936	819	
200	2400	480	720	1200	720	960	840	

Figure 14 - Calorie Table

How To Use the Calorie Table

1. Locate LBM in the first column and find your Lean Body Mass in pounds

2. Find your base calories. The amount of resting calories based on the LBM.

3. Locate the number of calories used during your type of work activity. Add this amount to your base calories. The total will be the amount of calories your body uses on an average day.

4. Find your type of training activity, then move down the column until you reach your LBM in pounds. Add the calories you use during training to the total of your base and work calories.

The following body composition evaluations will clarify this new approach to determining how many calories the body uses based on the Lean Body Mass.

Example 1:	**Example 2:**
Scale weight 110 lbs.	Scale weight 165 lbs.
LBM 90 lbs.	LBM 90 lbs.
Fat 20 lbs.	Fat 75 lbs.

Calories Used based on their LBM

Example 1:	**Example 2:**
Base Cal. 1080 cal.	Base Cal. 1080 cal.
Work Cal. 116 cal.	Work Cal. 116 cal.
Total Cal. 1196 cal.	Total Cal. 1196 cal.

Calories Used in One Hour of Training

Example 1:	**Example 2:**
65% - 85% T.H.R. 432 cal.	No training 0 cal.
Total from above 1196 cal.	Total from above 1196 cal.

Her Body Uses 1628 cal.	**Her Body Uses 1196 cal.**

Both women use the same base calories because their LBM is the same. If both women ate 1400 calories each day, the larger woman, would have an intake of 204 calories more than the 1196 calories her LBM uses. The 110 lb. woman who's LBM uses 1628 calories each day, will use 228 calories more than she eats.

Eating 1400 cal/day the larger woman would add a pound or two of fat to her body each month, because of her calorie excess each day. She is also, likely to lose muscle due to her inactivity. To lose fat and maintain her muscle mass, she has to eat at least 1000 calories each day. Her rate of change will be slow unless she does some type of training activity.

The 110 pound woman will lose approximately two pounds of fat each month eating 1400 cal/day. She could also eat 1600 cal/day, and maintain her weight.

How to Find Your Average Calories per Day

The average number of calories is very important when we begin to design an improvement program. The calories we require depends on our personal goals, Lean Mass and activity level. To determine the average number of calories we use per day, add the total number of calories used during one week and divide by seven.

Example: 110 pound woman (90 lbs LBM)

Day 1 - 1300 calories
Day 2 - 1700 calories
Day 3 - 1600 calories
Day 4 - 1800 calories

Day 5 - 1600 calories
Day 6 - 1800 calories
Day 7 - 2100 calories

Total - 11,900 calories/week

Average calories/day - 1700
The weekly total (11,900) divided by seven

Comparing the number of calories we eat per day to the number of calories the lean mass uses per day will determine our individual rate of improvement.

The first reaction to the total calories one uses in a day usually is: "I couldn't possibly use that many calories in a day. I'd get fat if I ate that much!" There is a tendency to think that a low calorie intake of 500 to 900 calories per day, is the only way to lose fat. Fat loss occurs consistently when the correct amount of protein, fat and carbohydrate calories is balanced with the individual's activity level.

Now that we understand the number of calories we use, it is important to choose how many calories we will eat each day based on our personal goals. Three types of goals are considered.

<u>Goal</u>	<u>Calorie Requirement</u>
Decrease body fat:	Eat 20% less calories than are used each day.
Increase lean mass:	Eat the same number of calories the LBM uses. 20% of these calories should be protein.
Maintain present weight and shape:	Eat the same number of calories the LBM uses.

The LBM determines how many calories we use during various activities. While it is important to balance calories to activity, it is just as important and much more fun to balance food to our activity. Calories are units of energy provided by food. Even though we *think* calories, we don't *eat* calories. We eat food! The next step is to learn how we can eat in order to control weight and shape, rather than *not* eat to lose weight.

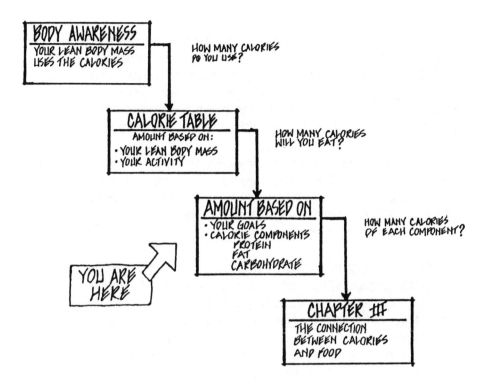

BODY AWARENESS
YOUR LEAN BODY MASS
USES THE CALORIES

HOW MANY CALORIES
DO YOU USE?

CALORIE TABLE
AMOUNT BASED ON:
• YOUR LEAN BODY MASS
• YOUR ACTIVITY

HOW MANY CALORIES
WILL YOU EAT?

AMOUNT BASED ON
• YOUR GOALS
• CALORIE COMPONENTS
  PROTEIN
  FAT
  CARBOHYDRATE

HOW MANY CALORIES
OF EACH COMPONENT?

YOU ARE
HERE

CHAPTER III
THE CONNECTION
BETWEEN CALORIES
AND FOOD

The Nature of Food

Our state of mind changes our concept and definition of food, moment by moment. When we are hungry, depressed, or in various states of emotion, thoughts and suggestions about food can certainly trigger our feelings. Most of us are controlled by food, rather than in control of our food. Have you ever noticed the difference between grocery shopping when you are famished, compared to shopping after you have eaten?

Food has a great influence on our body, energy level emotions, and productivity. Food can shape the body, dominate thoughts, control feelings, cause or relieve pain, create heart problems, or be the source of energy and vitality. Just as food can be the cause of many health concerns, food can also be the cure.

Our source of information regarding food comes from magazines, newspapers and television. The media's view of food is often designed for our mouths, minds and someone's profit, rather than our improved weight and shape. When based only on taste, convenience and diets, both the food and the information is incomplete.

The Lean Body Mass slowly deteriorates with incomplete food. Complete food means balancing proteins, fats and carbohydrates to the LBM. Wouldn't it be exciting if balancing food components to the Lean Body Mass meant eating more food?

All foods contain one or more of the main food components; proteins, fats or carbohydrates. Each component contains a specific number of calories. The body needs each component in the correct amount to accomplish our performance and appearance goals. Before learning the amounts, we will review what these components are, and how they are used.

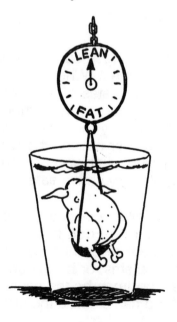

The Food Compostion Evaluation

Protein

Protein is the substance necessary for our body's growth and repair. During the growth process, Lean Body Mass tissues require a higher amount of protein. Once we have stopped growing, the body still continues to repair 24 hours a day, every day. The repair process requires that the components of protein (amino acids) are present in the bloodstream and are available to the tissues at all times.

When we have not consumed enough food rich in protein, the body will break down and use its own muscle tissue as a protein source. The amino acids in protein are necessary for the 6000 enzyme reactions that allow our body to function. They are also essential to the healing process after injury. Our bodies require *complete protein*, which means that all amino acids must be present.

Information about protein and its relationship to the LBM is not usually available to us in a format that can be used to improve. It is possible to find information about protein and still be confused about how much and what type of protein to eat. The confusion clears when protein is explained in a way that we can understand.

How Much: There are standard daily amounts of protein recommended by the government. These are called United States Recommended Daily Allowances (USRDA). The USRDA amounts for adults and children are the minimum amounts of protein required by our bodies each day. This standard amount may be inadequate for your protein needs. Your specific protein amount each day can be determined by using the standard requirements as a base and modifying the amount depending on your Lean Body Mass. (This will be discussed in Chapter Three.)

What Type Of Protein: Our usual sources of protein are animal, fowl, fish and seafood products. Proteins are made of amino acids, which also occur in plant sources such as wheat, legumes, nuts, seeds and soy products, to name a few. The most important difference between plant and other protein is the amino acid composition. The amino acid composition of protein determines whether it is complete or incomplete.

Complete protein is composed of 22 amino acids. Eight of the amino acids are called essential, which means they cannot be manufactured within our bodies and must be obtained from the food we eat. The remaining 14 amino acids can be manufactured within our bodies from other protein components. Foods of animal, fish or fowl origin do contain all essential amino acids, and therefore are a source of complete protein. Plant protein is lacking in one or more of the eight essential amino acids and therefore is an incomplete protein.

In the discussion of complete and incomplete proteins it is important to review the vegetarian style of eating. An increasing number of people are choosing a diet that eliminates most or all animal sources of protein. To obtain the daily protein requirement under these conditions, a proper combination of plant protein is necessary.

Vegetarianism

Vegetarians avoid or restrict food products of animal origin. The main concern when eating only plant protein is obtaining the essential amino acids. A vegetarian eating program can include the vital amino acids with proper food combining. My personal changes in LBM and fat during eighteen months as a vegetarian, and the body composition reports of other vegetarians, have led to the following conclusions:

- Properly combining plant protein is necessary for a vegetarian diet to supply the essential amino acids. People merely avoiding animal products experience an increase in fat and a decrease in LBM.

- Vegetarians tend to include seeds, nuts, and cheese to increase their protein, in reality these foods contain excessive fat and little protein.

Vegetarianism can be effective for weight and shape improvement with knowledge and planning. I encourage vegetarians to combine food for their protein requirements and monitor their eating program with regular body composition evaluations. Those of you interested in a vegetarian diet can obtain valuable information on a more complete approach from the book *Diet for a Small Planet*, by Frances M. Lappe.

Fats

There are two main types of fat: body fat and food fat. Body fat, for the most part, represents what we would like to change about our body. Food fat represents one of the tastes we like about our food. The relationship between the two, which is very simple and often overlooked, is that excess fat calories in our food causes excess fat on our bodies. In truth, our shape is not a random coincidence; it is a result!

With all of the information available regarding fat and its connection with cholesterol and heart disease, there is still very little awareness of how to use that data to affect the weight and shape of our body. The most important step in reducing the amount of fat in our diet is learning, first, how much fat we can use and, second, what type foods contain the fat.

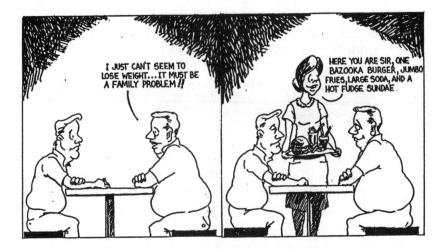

We think we "are" fat, we don't think we "eat" fat.

How Much Fat Can We Eat?

Our bodies can only use a small percentage of fat each meal and each day, depending on our LBM and activity level. There are more calories in fat than in protein or carbohydrates. One gram of fat has 9 calories while one gram of protein or carbohydrate has 4 calories.

The most valuable way to understand food fat is to learn what types of foods have a high fat content.

High fat foods come in many forms:

- Butter, sour cream, ice cream, avocados, french fries, cheeseburgers and pizza are a few.

- Egg yolks, salad dressings and oil.

- Most meats, fowl and some seafood contain fat.

- Nuts, seeds, peanut butter and cheese.

- Lard, refried beans, hot dogs, pastries and desserts.

Although fats are great for taste, fats are also concentrated calories. A small volume of fat contains a great number of calories. Therefore, the secret to reducing the fat on our bodies is to reduce the fat in our diet. Decreasing fat cannot happen unless we learn *how much* fat is present in the food we eat.

Carbohydrates

Carbohydrates are the primary energy source for all body functions and muscular performance. One of the main purposes of carbohydrates is to help control protein and fat metabolism. The presence of carbohydrates prevents the body from using muscle as an energy source, and allows us to use stored body fat.

1. Main function: to serve as fuel for energy.

   a. Energy from carbohydrates is used to power the muscles. Carbohydrates are the main food for energy level and performance.

   b. Carbohydrates are stored in the muscles and in the liver, in a form termed glycogen. Carbohydrates are also stored in the bloodstream, in a readily used form called glucose. Following a meal, excess carbohydrates are converted to, and stored as glycogen in the muscle and liver. Once the storage capacity is reached, the excess carbohydrates are partially eliminated and partially stored as fat. If you eat over the amount of calories your LBM is capable of using and don't exercise, you get fat. This process occurs even on a low fat diet.

2. Preserves Muscle Protein.

In the absence of carbohydrate, protein is used as the source of energy. Muscle protein can and will be eaten by the body for energy, if you don't eat your carbohydrates in the form of pasta, bread, potatoes, rice, and vegetables.

3. Metabolic primer.

Carbohydrates serve as a primer for fat metabolism. Certain food fragments from brokendown carbohydrates must be available in order to metabolize fat. Without carbohydrates, you cannot use the fat your body has stored. Physiologists have said, "Fat is burned in a carbohydrate flame."

4. Fuel for the nervous system.

Carbohydrates are essential for the proper operation of the brain and nervous system. The brain uses carbohydrates (glucose) as fuel, and does not have a stored fuel supply. When you stop eating carbohydrates, the body breaks down muscle protein to make carbohydrates to feed the brain.

Carbohydrate Balance in Exercise

Understanding the balance of carbohydrates in exercise is absolutely essential in achieving whatever level of weight, shape, and performance we desire.

Intense Exercise: hard running, biking, or skipping rope (65% - 85% Training Heart Rate)

1. When training hard, you use carbohydrates called glycogen from the muscles doing the work. When this supply is depleted, you use the carbohydrates called glucose carried in the blood stream.

2. If you are training your legs very hard over a period of time, you can totally deplete your supply of glycogen and glucose in those muscles. Your arm, back, shoulder and chest muscles will not supply any of their glycogen to the depleted leg muscles. Runners and bikers for example, can totally use their glycogen supply within their leg muscles, blood, and liver, and halt their performance, called "hitting the wall". Their other muscles still have an adequate glycogen supply.

3. During intense exercise the need for oxygen is often greater than the supply. Carbohydrate is the only nutrient that provides the energy when there is insufficient oxygen.

The main point: *Fat is not a fuel for intense exercise.* This is often a real surprise, in that most of us grew up believing the harder we exercised or trained the more fat we would burn.

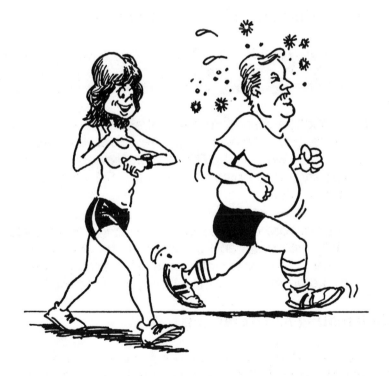

The Body Doesn't Burn Fat When You Work Harder

Moderate/ProlongedExercise: brisk walk or slow jog (50% - 60% Training Heart Rate)

1. You can use up to 50% carbohydrates for fuel, and increasing amounts of fat, with increased time. Meaning: exercise at a 50% to 60% (T.H.R.) burns more fat.

2. Do you ever get tired? Fatigue occurs when glycogen in the liver and specific muscles is depleted. Exercising at a moderate uses fat as fuel in addition to the glycogen from carbohydrates. This reduces fatigue.

3. You can participate in a moderately paced activity longer because it uses fat as fuel. Fat loss is a function of time, so the longer you exercise at a moderately active pace, the more fat you will burn.

What To Remember About Carbohydrates

- Carbohydrates are the main energy source for the body. They help preserve protein in the form of muscle tissue and allow fat to be used as energy.

- Carbohydrates have been of secondary importance in the American diet. However, the fact remains that our health and performance would benefit from consuming 50% to 75% complex carbohydrates.

- Carbohydrate digestion begins in the mouth, especially with grain and cereal starches. It then continues in the small intestines. This simply means, make an extra effort to chew your food well.

Undereating or Overeating

The Lean Body Mass requires a certain number of calories per day depending on our activities. There is also a specific amount of proteins, fats and carbohydrates needed to balance the daily calories. When the body's needs are satisfied, random eating patterns are eliminated.

Undereaters

Some people feel the calories listed in the calorie table are too high to achieve fat loss. With the calorie table based on Lean Body Mass, the importance of muscle tissue, and how the body needs fuel still fresh in your mind, let's review undereating.

Each person's body has a requirement for a certain number of calories per day. One of the basic rules is that the calorie requirement cannot be changed without a consequence. If fuel, in the form of food, is not provided, the body will initially use its own Lean Body Mass and small amounts of fat to provide the necessary energy. Later, within a few weeks, the activity and energy level will drop to match the food intake. On a short-term basis, if the calorie intake is not adequate the person will demonstrate the results of undereating in a number of ways:

- The blood sugar level drops.

- There is increased irritability.

- The activity and energy level decreases.

- There is an increase in percent of body fat, with an eventual decrease in the Lean Body Mass.

After reviewing cases and working with people, it is clear that undereaters have a difficult time *losing fat*, yet find it easy to *lose weight* according to the scale. Weight loss on the scale doesn't necessarily mean fat loss from your body. Weight loss can be composed of 40% to 60% Lean Body Mass. A high percentage of the remaining loss is water, and a low percentage is fat.

All types of undereaters have great difficulty with weight and shape control. By Lean Body Mass standards, a woman would be classified as an undereater if, her calorie requirement was 1600 calories used per day, and she:

1. Ate 900 calories per day, or less, in the correct proportion of proteins, fats and carbohydrates. (An excellent rule to follow is not to go below your resting calorie requirement per day in food consumption.)

2. Ate 1600 calories per day in correct proportions of proteins, fats and carbohydrates, all in one meal. The body needs a constant supply of nutrients throughout the day. For example, the body repairs itself 24 hours a day and sees this as overeating for one meal and undereating until the next day.

3. Under-ate protein, but ate 1600 calories in fat and carbohydrates. The body has specific requirements for the major food elements: proteins, carbohydrates and fats. The body views this as undereating, and would use muscle to supply the necessary protein.

4. Ate 1600 calories per day and under-ate in terms of food value. In other words, she ate all processed and refined foods. We will not deal in depth with the importance of vitamins and minerals. However, these food elements are absolutely essential for the more than 6000 chemical reactions necessary for body processes to continue. Because much of the food we eat is processed and overcooked, it is worth considering vitamin/mineral supplements.

5. Ate excessive protein and fat and under-ate carbohydrates. Carbohydrates present in the body are essential for muscle and brain fuel. Inadequate carbohydrate consumption is a guarantee that your body will use muscle tissue to supply the carbohydrates you are not eating.

Overeaters

Overeaters are an interesting group. I have talked with these people, read behavior modification studies, psychologists' and psychiatrists' case history reports, and have come to one conclusion: The person overeats the wrong foods and undereats the necessary foods. The overeater is really an undereater who overeats calories and undereats in food value.

The overeating is done with fats and refined carbohydrates. These foods have more calories for each amount of food, and minimal nutritional value. Fat has nine calories per gram. An example would be a commercial muffin, which could have 350 to 400 calories, compared to a home-baked muffin containing 200 calories, The difference is in the hidden amount of oil and butter.

Overeating is rarely done with necessary foods, such as protein or properly-prepared complex carbohydrates. When was the last time you heard of a person overeating steamed broccoli, or stuffing themselves with baked halibut and baked potatoes? A person usually overeats high fat and refined foods, such as desserts, while the complex carbohydrates and proteins are not being eaten. The point is: The overeater is actually undereating the necessary foods.

In our society, we somehow are convinced that if a solution is not complicated, expensive, and presented to us by a doctor, it cannot possibly work. The cure to undereating or overeating is to eat the correct amount of protein, fats and carbohydrates for your Lean Body Mass. If you choose to overeat, then follow this general program. After satisfying the calorie requirements of your Lean Body Mass with proteins, fats and carbohydrates, eat as much refined sugars and fats as you would like, to satisfy your mouth. This is much better than eating an entire meal of fat and sugars, and undereating in terms of food value.

When people satisfy their basic requirements first and then overeat, a strange phenomena occurs within a relatively short time. The correct proportion of proteins, fats and carbohydrates begins to be so satisfying, that the person eats less of the unnecessary foods.

When the person eats a balance of complex carbohydrates and protein, three changes occur:

1. The blood sugar level remains stable.

2. Cravings and the tendency to binge are eliminated.

3. Mood swings disappear. The person becomes more emotionally stable.

Wrapping Up

Calorie and food composition has played a major role in what has happened to your body in the past, and will have complete influence over what will happen to your body in the future. As you proceed to Chapter 3, remember these points:

- The muscle portion of your Lean Body Mass shapes your body and uses stored body fat.

- Protein is necessary for muscle growth, repair, and maintenance.

- Carbohydrates are muscle and brain fuel.

- Stored body fat can provide fuel for our muscles to function, under certain conditions.

- How much fuel we use per day is measured in calories. The number of calories used depends upon our Lean Body Mass in pounds and how active we are in both work and exercise.

- Once we know the calories we use per day, we can begin to plan our individual food program and determine how many calories we need.

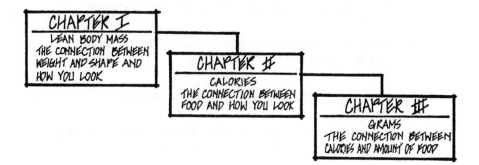

CHAPTER 3

The Missing Connection

*"The answers we want may be hidden
by the answers we know!"*

Overview

Our culture constantly struggles with weight and shape. Have you noticed the same difficulty occurs in our relationship with food? We all know there is a relationship between food and our bodies, and yet the connection continues to elude and confuse us. We continue to search and experiment with different diets, because the main link between food and our weight and shape has been overlooked. When the missing relationship is recognized and put into place, changes in your body's appearance are assured. These changes come from always being able to balance food to your activity level and goals.

The traditional approach, and I believe the reason for the ongoing confusion, is that we have all been trained to think that calories are the main link between food and our bodies. This has led to the belief that if we manage calories we will manage food; and, therefore, we are in control of our weight. Thinking "calories = food" is not wrong; it is incomplete. Using only calories as the foundation for our weight control program and the amount of food we eat is similar to making our decision about ideal weight by using the traditional bathroom scale. The point is that neither the bathroom scale nor calories can provide us with complete information.

Calories are necessary as a starting point. What's missing is how to convert calories into the right amount of food according to our Lean Body Mass. The power to control your weight and shape comes from an understanding of this missing portion. Chapter Three is designed to bring clarity to the connection between food and your body.

The Calorie Connection

After spending the last chapter converting Lean Body Mass to calories, we can say that using calories based on our LBM is an accurate place to start. Perhaps it is how we perceive calories that stops us from recognizing what keeps us from improving our weight and shape. "Calorie" is one word we have heard, seen and talked about for so long that it is often used without understanding. It is so much a part of our language and thinking that we have begun to believe that calories are things, and have lost sight of the fact that calories are energy and only exist after food is processed in the body.

The Traditional Approach

The ongoing problem with our weight, shape and food could be summarized as follows: We "know" that altering calories does change our body, even though it never seems to be the result we want, and it never seems to last. Also, we seem to get a little more out of shape every year. At some point, we begin to wonder if the best we can hope for is that the deterioration process will slow down. We also know this process has something to do with food. It is quite possible that the answers we *want* are hidden by the answers we *know*.

The obvious connection between food and our bodies is calories. Using calories as the basis for establishing weight and shape control programs leads to one of two possible beliefs:

Belief #1: Calories are food.

Belief #2: Calories come from the protein, fat and carbohydrate components in the food.

Belief #1: Calories Are Food.

The first question that comes to mind when we want to improve our weight is, "How much food?" Most of us grew up with the concept that calories are the same as food. The reasoning is, calories are food; food makes us fat; and so we will simply eat fewer calories. In everyday terms that means: "Eat whatever we want, only less of it!"

To reduce calories, we simply have a bag of Doritos and an apple for lunch, or a salad instead of a meal. We develop creative ways to reduce food without any concept of what kind of food, and how much reduction, would be best. The amount of food reduction depends upon the urgency of the situation; in other words; how soon is the class reunion?

Results From Belief #1: The result of food restriction is that the lost weight returns, and any improvement in shape is short lived. Then our thought process becomes: Having low-calorie lunches more often during the week, and maybe skipping lunch or dinner altogether, might be better. All of this means more food restriction. The result of less food is loss of LBM, increasing fat and a reduced ability to burn the fat you already have. At some point in time, it occurs to us that just decreasing calories is not the complete answer.

Belief #2: Calories come from proteins, fats and carbohydrates.

In the first example, we believed that calories equaled food. In this example, we now believe that calories equal one of the food components. To reduce calories, simply reduce or eliminate one or more of these food components. The process of restriction, or even elimination of one of these three components, follows the same pattern and is the basis for most diet and food plans.

The problem with using a restrictive diet plan of fat, protein or carbohydrates is that we "know" that we have now found the answer. To understand the difference between food components, and begin to eliminate one of them to improve our body, makes great sense to our mind. However, our body's lean mass does not understand the process in the same way as our minds. The Lean Body Mass knows it needs a certain balance, or a percentage of proteins, fats and carbohydrates. Therefore, the minute we restrict one of these components, there is no possibility of a balance for the body.

Result From Belief #2: The results in weight and shape are similar to the Belief #1, due to an imbalanced reduction of the protein, fat and carbohydrate amounts. When a particular low carbohydrate or low protein diet plan is not working, we immediately assume this was not the right plan for us, and find another program. At some point we learn that an imbalanced restriction of a food component doesn't work. Knowing this allows us to focus on the balance of proteins, fats and carbohydrates. Then we have the real truth: eat the right percent of each food component.

While our beliefs may not be the answer, they provide us a way of discovering what doesn't work. As a result, we are now able to pursue a better answer about weight and shape. The most effective way to improve weight and shape is *with* food. Using food requires starting with calories.

Knowing our personal calorie needs is not the answer, it is the starting point, like a ticket to get in the gate. The next step is to convert calories into the amount of proteins, fats and carbohydrates that will fit our weight and shape goals.

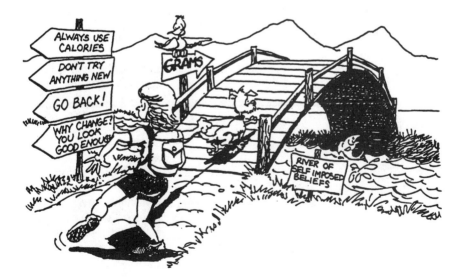

How Many Calories Will You Eat?

The number of calories you eat per day depends upon your goals for weight and shape. Regardless of how specific your goals are for changing performance or developing a particular body, the bottom line is always in the category of losing fat or gaining lean mass.

The calories we use per day, from the Calorie Table (Chapter 2, p. 61), is determined by our LBM and activity level. The objective now is to clarify our goals, determine our best number of calories per day, and convert those calories into food that fits our personal program.

What goal do you choose for your body?

Current Lean Body Mass in pounds   _____   Future: _____
Current fat mass in pounds   _____   Future: _____

Choice	LBM	Fat	Basic Program
1	Maintain	Decrease	Eat less calories plus aerobic training
2	Increase	Decrease	Eat slightly less calories. Include resistance and aerobic training
3	Increase	Maintain	Maintain calories and increase resistance training.
4	Maintain	Maintain	When you are pleased with your evaluation, maintain your present program.

Once you have determined the number of calories you use each day, how many calories to eat will be made on the basis of one of three possible goals:

1. Maintain Present Weight and Shape:

Eat the same number of calories your body uses per day.

2. Lose Body Fat:

The general fat loss rule is to eat less calories than you use per day. Eating less food is a delicate subject because most people insist on drastically undereating to accomplish their goals faster. Undereating doesn't work!

A 20% reduction of the daily calories is the best place to start. Be certain to stay above your base calories. For example: if your body uses 1400 calories per day, a 20% reduction means you eat approximately 1100 calories per day.

3. Gain Lean Mass:

To gain weight simply consume the same calories you use per day, and be certain 20% of the calories are from protein. Gaining weight does not necessarily mean gaining size. Consider this program when you weight train under supervision, have the discipline to stick to your schedule, and have a body composition evaluation every two to four weeks.

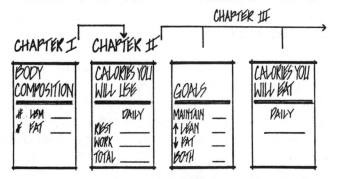

Figure 15 - Update of Your Goals and Program

From Calories to Food

The three major food components provide fuel for energy and substance for growth and repair. There is not one formula for proteins, carbohydrates and fats that will fit all people. There is a range for each component that provides what we all want: the ability to control our weight and shape. Before choosing the percentage of each component for your initial program, we will review proteins, fats and carbohydrates and their purposes:

1. Dietary Protein is necessary for growth and repair. Three small protein servings per day will provide a 24 hour protein supply to the body. When dietary protein is not present, the muscle tissue is broken down to supply the necessary protein components (amino acids). Extra dietary protein, beyond the correct amount for that meal, is partially eliminated and partially stored as fat.

2. Dietary Fats are necessary only in small amounts. Extra fat is treated the same as extra protein. It is partially eliminated and partly stored as fat.

3. Dietary Carbohydrates are the main energy source for the Lean Body Mass. They are also a protection system for muscle protein. They initiate fat breakdown, are fuel for the brain, and are a source of fiber. Extra carbohydrates, like proteins and fats, are both eliminated and stored in the body as fat.

We have learned that overeating proteins, fats and carbohydrates causes fat and that undereating causes a loss of lean mass. This would clearly indicate that eating the "right" amount of each component is important. The question is: What amount is right? The right amount fits within a range, and the specific answer depends upon our LBM, activity level and our goals.

With this as background, and knowing that the majority of people are quite dissatisfied with their body and its performance, let's examine how traditional food percentages or proportions would contribute to the problem. The average American appears to have two distinct eating styles.

Standard American Diet #1

Protein	30-35%
Fats	35-50%
Carbohydrates	25-50%

In this example there is an excess of protein, and a 10% to 40% excess of fat calories, which certainly adds to body fat. Under-eating 10% to 25% in carbohydrates guarantees the loss of lean mass over the months and years. Using this diet, it is possible for a person to eat the exact number of calories he or she needs per day. However, if those calories are consumed in the above percentages, this person's body will gain fat. Even worse, this person may never realize why.

Standard American Diet #2

Protein	5-10%
Fats	25%
Carbohydrates	70%

These percentages are further complicated by the fact that these people, mostly women, have learned to control their weight by undereating. Consuming less than your base calories per day is a sure way to lose Lean Body Mass. There are not enough amino acids for body processes and repair with only 5% of the food eaten being protein. Therefore the body will break down its existing body tissue for the necessary amino acids.

These people are generally under-muscled and inactive. A dietary fat intake of 25% is too high for their activity level, which results in an increase of body fat. A diet of 70% carbohydrates may be appropriate, depending on their activity level.

If our typical eating pattern leads to a decrease of muscle and an increase of body fat, it should be no surprise that many of us are out of shape, fat, and under-muscled. This includes children and teenagers, as well as adults. The common solution to weight and shape problems is to eat less, fast, skip meals, and then over-eat. This is always done with the same unbalanced percentages of proteins, fats and carbohydrates.

Examining our standard eating programs has proven which percentages we *don't* want to use. Using your Lean Body Mass, you can find the balance of food you need for your body. After eliminating the percentages that don't work, what remains is the range of percentages for proteins, fats and carbohydrates that can be adapted to your individual body.

Recomended Percentages

Protein	15-25%
Fat	10-25%
Carbohydrates	50-75%

At this point, you may begin to realize, for the first time, why other food programs have never created lasting results. Now, the next step is to select the component percentage to use for your initial program.

Which Percentages are Best for You?

The optimum percentage for each food component will fit within the recommended range for each of us. There is a fairly wide range for each component. This will allow you to choose a program that is most like your present eating style, and that you can work with from the beginning. There are different plans. Therefore, you can change your percentages at any time.

If a person is used to eating excess protein and fat, I advise a 25% protein, 25% fat and 50% carbohydrate plan for the first six weeks. This is called Plan I. After the initial adjustment, four to eight weeks the person is encouraged to alter the percentages in this way:

Plan		Protein	Fat	Carbohydrates
I	1st 6 weeks	25%	25%	50%
II	2nd 6 weeks	25%	20%	55%
III	3rd 6 weeks	20%	20%	60%
IV	4th 6 weeks	20%	15%	65%

Figure 16 - Percentage Plans

Which plan will you use initially? One recommendation is to choose the plan which most closely matches your current protein percentage intake. Indicate your choice by simply underlining or circling one of the above plans. It is not necessary to start with Plan I. Begin with the plan you feel will be the most comfortable.

Experimenting with different percentage plans at six week intervals will allow you to find the plan that best suits you. The percentage plans are ultimately a personal choice. Each plan will have an effect on your body composition and shape. I have not found positive results outside these percentages.

Some clients find they prefer Plan II; and yet Plan IV would create better results from a body composition standpoint. Other clients are pleased with their improvements on Plan I and elect to stay at these percentages.

These plans are a way to improve your body composition by adjusting the percent of food components. These plans put you in control.

Let's review the reasoning for working with percentage amounts of food components:

1. Your Lean Body Mass, not your total weight, uses the calories and needs a specific amount of protein, fats and carbohydrates.

2. Your most rapid improvement will be with one of the listed percentage plans. Eating programs that do not balance food components with activity and Lean Body Mass, will not work for human bodies.

3. Undereating or overeating certain components, such as eliminating fat completely, increasing carbohydrates, or any other creative combination outside of these percentage amounts, will result in decreasing lean mass, increasing fat, or both.

4. As your LBM or activity level changes, you can easily alter the percentage of food components to match these changes.

It is useful to list the total calories you will eat, the percent of each component, and the calories from each food before proceeding to the next step.

Your Total Calories per Day: _____

Protein:	____% equals	____calories/day
Carbohydrate:	____% equals	____calories/day
Fat:	____% equals	____calories/day

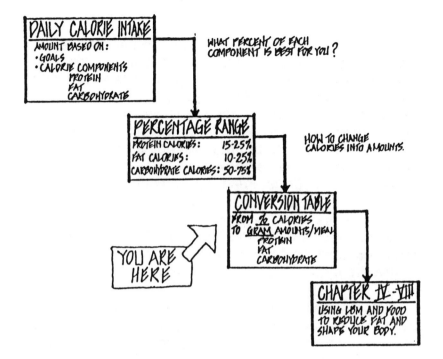

Grams

In our search for the missing connection between food and our bodies, we have reviewed both the limitation and the importance of using calories. The next step is to convert your percentage of protein, fat and carbohydrate calories into gram amounts. It is actually the gram measurement for each food component that is the missing link between calories, food and our body. Grams are the standard measurements for the fat, protein and carbohydrate amounts in foods. For example:

Food		amount in grams		
amount in ounces	Cal	Pro	Fat	Carb
3-1/2 oz. roasted chicken light meat, skinless	166	31.5	3.4	0.0
3-1/2 oz. baked potato	93	2.6	0.1	21.1

If the percentage of protein you need per meal is measured in calories, a formula and calculation is necessary to determine how many ounces of chicken to eat. If your protein per meal is measured in grams, the Composition of Foods Table (Appendix B) clearly lists how many ounces of a food contain the protein you need. We can look up the grams of protein in any food we choose, and at the same time see how many grams of fat and grams of carbohydrate are in this particular food.

Once we know the gram amount of proteins, fats and carbohydrates we need each meal, we become aware of food content labels and begin looking for fat grams in our favorite foods. This is a key to your ongoing success.

Using grams makes it easier to select our foods because protein, fat and carbohydrate amounts are listed in grams. The conversion from your percentage of calories to grams has already been done for you in the Gram Conversion tables. (pp. 97 - 99) This conversion is only on paper. It will serve you best when you make the conversion from calories to grams in your own thinking. In other words, to make this work, you need to think about food and food components in terms of grams.

"Thinking" grams instead of calories gives you the ability to provide your Lean Body Mass with fuel in the right percentage at any time and anywhere. When you are hungry and need food, you find the closest and most convenient food supply. The saying is: "You see what you know." When you know only calories, your choices are limited and the results are negative in from a body composition standpoint.

If we know more--such as 20 grams of protein, 60 grams of carbohydrates and 10 grams of fat--we find the closest food supply that will provide the necessary amount.

Once the right percentages are selected, there is no longer a need to refer to calories. You can now think and talk in terms of how many grams of each food component you need per meal. Once you are familiar with grams, it will take only a matter of seconds for you to determine the grams you need each meal, from your Lean Body Mass. After a few meals, there will be an instant conversion from protein, fat and carbohydrate grams into the "right" amounts of your favorite foods.

Grams are the real connection between food and your body. Thinking and conversing in terms of grams is actually a new language. Once learned, this "language" is easier and more accurate than calories.

Please review the charts on the following pages, which indicate the number of grams per day and grams per meal of each food component at different percentages. At this point, you may be saying, "This is too much detail about grams, and I still don't know how this will fit into my next meal of mashed potatoes and gravy." Your starting point is to use your favorite food to find what percentage of proteins, fats and carbohydrates works best. I can assure you that in the next section of this book we will turn the grams into something very real, tasty and fun to eat.

Update of Your Goal and Program

The steps in your program up to this point are represented in the map on the following page. Indicate your results and choices in the spaces provided.

We will assume at this point that you eat, or will now consider eating, three meals each day. It is best to know what the Lean Body Mass needs and play by the body's rules rather than to think your body uses protein or carbohydrates only when you decide to provide these substances.

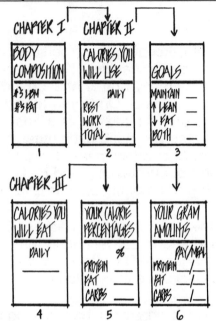

Figure 17 - Update of Your Goals and Program

1. Indicate your present pounds of *Lean Body Mass and fat* from your latest body composition evaluation.

2. Indicate the number of *calories you use*, determined from the Calorie Table (Chapter 2, p. 61), by your Lean Body Mass and activity level

3. Choose how you will change your body and indicate *your goal* in the third box. The choices are: maintain, increase lean mass, decrease fat, or both.

4. Indicate the number of *calories you will eat* per day depending upon your goals. (Figure 15, p. 87)

5. Choose the percentage plan for your first six week program (Figure 16, p. 91), and indicate the *percentages* of protein, fat and carbohydrates

6. Use the calorie to gram conversion tables, (Figures 18 - 20, pp. 97 - 99) to determine the number of protein, fat and carbohydrate *grams you will eat*.

PROTEIN CONVERSION TABLE

CALORIE PERCENTAGE TO GRAMS

CALORIES PER DAY	GRAMS PROTEIN PER DAY			GRAMS PROTEIN PER MEAL		
	25%	20%	15%	25%	20%	15%
800	50	40	30	17	13	10
900	57	45	34	19	15	11.5
1000	63	50	38	21	17	13
1200	75	60	45	25	20	15
1400	88	70	53	29	24	18
1600	100	80	60	34	27	20
1800	113	90	68	38	30	23
2000	126	100	76	42	34	26
2200	138	110	83	46	37	28
2400	150	120	90	50	40	30
2600	163	130	98	54	44	33
2800	176	140	106	58	48	36
3000	189	150	114	63	51	38
3200	200	160	120	68	54	40
3400	213	170	128	72	57	43
3600	226	180	136	76	60	46
3800	238	190	143	80	64	48
4000	252	200	152	84	68	52

Figure 18 - Protein Conversion Table

Directions:

1. Find the calories you will eat each day in the left-hand vertical column.

2. Move across to the percentage of protein you chose from the percentage plans (Figure 16, p. 91). Indicate this amount as your gram amount per/meal for protein. (step six, Figure 17, p. 96)

3. Move further to the same percentage, and indicate this number as your grams of protein per/day in step six.

FAT CONVERSION TABLES

CALORIE PERCENTAGE TO GRAMS

CALORIES PER DAY	GRAMS FAT PER DAY				GRAMS FAT PER MEAL			
	25%	20%	15%	10%	25%	20%	15%	10%
800	22	18	14	8	7	6	4.5	3
900	25	20	15.5	9.5	8	6.5	5	3.5
1000	28	22	17	11	9	7	5.5	4
1200	33	27	20	13	11	9	7	4.5
1400	39	31	23	16	13	10	8	5
1600	44	36	27	18	15	12	9	6
1800	50	40	30	20	17	13	10	7
2000	56	44	33	22	19	15	11	7.5
2200	61	49	37	25	20	16	12	8
2400	67	53	40	27	22	18	13	9
2600	72	58	43	29	24	19	14	10
2800	78	62	47	31	26	21	16	10.5
3000	83	67	50	33	28	22	17	11
3200	89	71	53	35	30	24	18	12
3400	94	75.5	57	38	31	25	19	12.5
3600	100	80	60	40	33	27	20	13
3800	105.5	84	63	42	35	28	21	14
4000	111	89	67	44	37	30	22	15

Figure 19 - Fat Conversion Table

Directions:

1. Find the calories you will eat each day in the left-hand vertical column.

2. Move across to the percentage of protein you chose from the percentage plans (Figure 16, p. 91). Indicate this amount as your gram amount per/meal for protein. (step six, Figure 17, p. 96)

3. Move further to the same percentage, and indicate this number as your grams of protein per/day in step six.

CARBOHYDRATE CONVERSION TABLE

CALORIE PERCENTAGE TO GRAMS

CALORIES PER DAY	GRAMS CARBOHYDRATES PER DAY					GRAMS CARBOHYDRATES PER MEAL				
	50%	55%	60%	65%	70%	50%	55%	60%	65%	70%
800	100	110	120	130	140	33	37	40	43	47
900	112.5	124	135	146.5	157.5	37.5	41.5	45	48.5	53
1000	125	138	150	163	175	42	46	50	54	59
1200	150	165	180	195	210	50	55	60	65	70
1400	175	193	210	228	245	59	64	70	76	82
1600	200	220	240	260	280	67	74	80	87	94
1800	225	248	270	293	315	75	83	90	98	105
2000	250	276	300	326	350	84	92	100	108	118
2200	275	303	330	358	285	92	101	110	119	129
2400	300	330	360	390	420	100	110	120	130	140
2600	325	358	390	423	455	109	120	130	141	152
2800	350	386	420	456	490	118	128	140	152	164
3000	375	413	450	488	525	125	138	150	163	175
3200	400	440	480	520	560	134	148	160	174	188
3400	425	468	510	553	595	142	156	170	184	199
3600	450	496	540	586	630	150	165	180	195	210
3800	475	524	570	619	665	158	175	190	206	222
4000	500	550	600	650	700	167	183	200	217	233

Figure 20 - Carbohydrate Conversion Table

Directions:

1. Find the calories you will eat each day in the left-hand vertical column.

2. Move across to the percentage of protein you chose from the percentage plans (Figure 16, p. 91). Indicate this amount as your gram amount per/meal for protein. (step six, Figure 17, p. 96)

3. Move further to the same percentage, and indicate this number as your grams of protein per/day in step six.

Wrapping Up

The Lean Body Mass is the part of the body that uses energy to perform and stay alive. This energy comes from food and the measurement of this energy is called calories. Calories come from the proteins, fats, and carbohydrates in food. In reality, a calorie does not exist until a particle of food is used in the body. What we need to know is:

1. How many calories does the body need per day?

2. What percentage of these calories comes from proteins, fats, and carbohydrates?

3. How much food does that percentage equal in grams? A gram of each food component is worth so many calories of energy. The calorie conversion to grams for the food components are:

1 gram of protein =	4 calories
1 gram of carbohydrate =	4 calories
1 gram of fat =	9 calories

It is important to know how many grams of each food component are in the food we eat. From the amounts we can determine whether or not the food will support us in obtaining our goal. For example, which of the following foods would support you best.

- 3-1/2 ounces of low-fat cottage cheese has 14 grams of protein and two grams of fat.

- 3-1/2 ounces of peanut butter has 27 grams of protein and 49 grams of fat.

The specific grams your body needs each day and each meal are calculated for you in the protein, fat and carbohydrate intake charts. These amounts are based on how many calories the Lean Body Mass uses each day. Since the human body cannot create protein from carbohydrates and fats, it is essential that we eat the correct grams of protein each meal.

The issue of food, body weight and shape would be less complicated if people ate a certain number of grams of each food component each meal, and then used a body composition report to find out what results that combination of food provides. By using grams we can start to get a sense of the amounts and proportions needed, and then easily convert this into food we like.

The first three chapters provided new information and the various tables to work with the new data. These beginning chapters have added to what you know. Knowing may be enough in itself; or you may choose to implement what you know. Rather than a "have-to-do" approach to dieting, this approach is a process of awareness, which will direct the daily choices you make about shopping, cooking, eating and training.

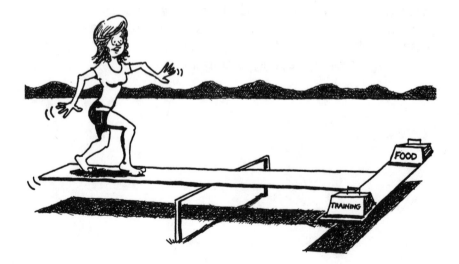

**Balancing food and training to your Lean Body Mass
is easier than it seems.**

CHAPTER 4

Creating A Relationship With Training

"The results of training are consistent--food allows the results to be visible or hidden."

Overview

With information about your body and about your food program as background, you are ready for the part of your personalized program called Action. This is not an answer to "What should I do?" It is more an answer to "What result do I want?" Your physical self--weight and shape--is, and always has been, the result of your food and activity. Your body is like a mirror that reveals whether or not your eating and training activities are in balance. Regardless of the reasons and excuses people give for their present weight and shape, the body is ready at all times to respond consistently and accurately to any food and training program.

The purpose of this chapter is not to play "follow the leader" with other exercise books. We could fill rooms with what has been said about training and exercise.

Our purpose is to develop a context--a way of "thinking" training and "talking" training--that encourages each of us to become experts regarding our own body.

What Is Training?

Let's examine a new way to define training. If the definition is accurate, it will serve you well in any circumstance, and will be a solid foundation from which to make your choices about your body, food and activities. Training means the type of activity that maintains or increases muscle and decreases fat. Body composition monitoring helps us learn if our "training" is producing the result we want. This definition eliminates the "right/wrong" opinions about different training activities, and has us focus on the results we are getting on our body composition reports. Training carries one absolute guarantee:

**The results of training are consistent, and
food allows those results to be visible.**

An improper balance of food and training can cancel the best weight and shape programs. There seems to be much controversy about the balance of food to activity, and about which program to use. The controversy appears to lie in the discrepancy or imbalance between our opinions, which we call Human Traits, and the natural course of events, which we call Natural Laws. The following examples will demonstrate how human traits may be a barrier to our progress.

Human Trait #1

"I can lose five pounds of fat in three days by not eating--I've done it before."

Natural Law #1

There are 3500 calories in one pound of fat. If your body uses 300 calories per hour during training, and one-half of these calories are fat, it will take approximately 24 one-hour sessions to use one pound of fat.

Human Trait #2

"I exercise as hard as I can every day and never seem to make any progress."

Natural Law #2

The human body burns fat more efficiently at a slower training heart rate.

Human Trait #3

"All the women on my side of the family carry their extra weight on their hips and thighs and there is nothing we can do to change a family pattern!"

Natural Law #3

The most inactive part of our body stores the fat with no regard for other family members.

The balance or the imbalance that exists between food and training changes our body. Using human traits and beliefs as the basis for a training program ends in frustration, futility and no change. Using the body's natural laws as the basis of our personal training program allows great opportunities for change.

Will Training Work?

Your body assumes the shape of your activity. The body of a athlete assumes a shape for each particular event. These are consistent, high-level athletes, not someone with a casual weekend interest. The shoulder development of basketball players and swimmers, the leg development of bikers and speed skaters, and the body development of runners and cross-country skiers are all examples of how the body adapts to an activity.

The body also assumes the shape of inactivity. Different activities create variations in body shape while inactivity creates the same shape! The shape of inactivity is consistent. Our muscle memory systems are very efficient; and we can even get more efficient at inactivity. My point is, people provide an abundance of explanations and excuses about why their bodies look the way they do, their shape which results from inactivity or activity speaks louder than their words.

Your Body Doesn't Lie

Before starting a training program people frequently ask, "How do I know that a food and training program will work for me?" The answer is, "Your program is working perfectly for you at the present time!" Our body weight, shape and performance level are the result of what we have done with food and activity up to this point. To have a different result requires a change in what we are doing. The problem is that not many of us know how to change our training, food or time schedule to get the result we want.

To accomplish our goal for weight, shape and performance, we have the following resources: food, training (exercise), or both. The most efficient rate of improvement stems from a change in both food and training. Using muscle to eliminate fat and change your shape requires a degree of activity. Excess fat is lost when you use the muscle and train at a certain heart rate. The people sitting in a sauna to lose fat will be surprised to find their weight loss is water.

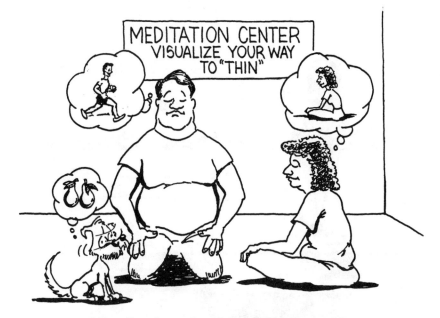

**"Visualize the action that creates the result,
as well as, the result itself."**

People who use meditation or positive image classes will be shocked to find that fat is not being dissolved through visualization only. Meditation and visualization are excellent supplements to a regular food and training program. In order to lose fat, a person's muscles must be in action.

The Relationship Between Training and the Body

Some people think dieting is the best method to improve weight and shape, while others are certain training is the best method. Consistent Body Composition Evaluations have proven that people using just exercise or just food showed very little change, and no lasting change, in their weight and shape. The true accomplishment in improving body composition comes from a balance between food and training. Using this balance, as it relates to Lean Body Mass, will allow a lifetime of control and will create the physical shape and energy you want.

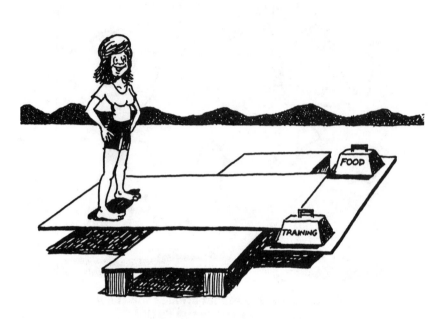

"Information creates a stable foundation from which you can comfortably change your body."

One of the major principles of the food/training balance is that the body operates according to the answers to two questions:

1. Is there enough activity to maintain or create an increase in Lean Body Mass?

2. Is there enough fuel for the activity?

We have a minimum activity level which maintains muscle tissue. Anything less than this level is termed "inactivity" by the muscle. People will often say, "Certainly, I'm training. I run from one end of the house to the other after these kids all day; and I'm exhausted." This activity qualifies as being busy, not training. Remember, training is an activity that maintains or increases your muscle, and decreases your fat.

Overtraining, on the other hand, is training without enough food to fuel the activity. This happens when people attempt to take shortcuts (human trait) and ignore how much fuel the body needs (natural law). These people consistently undereat and then train for faster results. According to the Lean Body Mass, there is not enough fuel for the amount of activity.

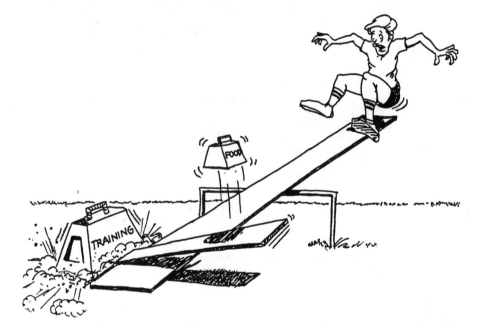

"In the beginning we may experience overtraining or undereating."

A more common situation is "no training". In this situation, no balance can exist between food and training, because there is not a way to counteract the lack of activity with less, or no, food. People who avoid training will decrease their food intake to balance the lack of activity. Ultimately the result is a loss of lean mass, and an increase of body fat. This is definitely a human trait which breaks every conceivable natural law related to the body.

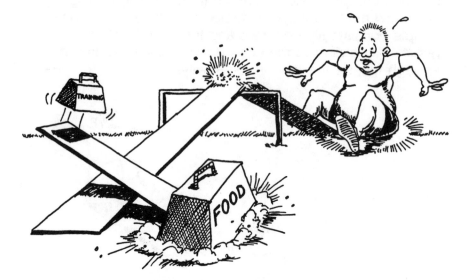

"A common pattern is overeating or undertraining."

Even though we know training is important, most of us, at some time, need an additional degree of motivation to inspire a new relationship with training.

Creating a Powerful Relationship with Training

Let's examine why our training plans might be defeated before we start, and then create a personal approach that fits each individual.

The mechanism that stops our training is usually hidden behind a number of complaints and excuses. Listen to what most people say about past and present training programs:

- "It didn't work anyway."

- "I just lost interest."

- "It was uncomfortable."

- "I didn't have anyone to train with."

- "Training is inconvenient."

- "My schedule doesn't allow it."

- "I was busy, tired, needed a break; and in general, it just wasn't any fun."

The above reasons for not training are used to justify why the person is no longer active. It is a challenge to create reasons for training when we believe this type of activity gets in the way of our main priorities. In this frame of mind, school becomes an interruption of summer and other vacations, while work becomes an inconvenience that happens between weekends, coffee breaks and 5 o'clock quitting time.

It is no wonder that training is seen as a chore or something we should do, instead of something that creates and takes care of the alive part of us--the Lean Body Mass. There is a strong possibility that no one ever created an opportunity for us to consider training as a possible access to energy, life, aliveness, shape, appearance, and fun.

What would it be like if at an early age, or even at our present age, we could develop a new approach to our Lean Body Mass and training that would shape our future selves? Here is a thought that may contribute to a new attitude about training.

Regardless of age, activity, or income, the muscle of your Lean Body Mass is the highest quality available! What would an athlete, or someone you call a performer, do with your muscle tissue? Let's be more specific. Which performer do you admire most? A skater, a dancer, a gymnast? Could you ever aspire to be that person? The answer is usually "absolutely not."

Most people describe these superb athletes as using every muscle cell 100%, in a way that develops and expresses their physical potential. Therefore, if we could give your body to such an athlete, he or she would develop 100% of your body's physical expression. An athlete is very much like the muscle. An athlete thinks in terms of maximum expression of potential; and muscle responds in terms of maximum expression of potential.

Your muscles expand and contract in perfect harmony with your food and training, just like the muscles of the athlete. If the athlete could have your muscles and develop their potential, why couldn't you? Why wouldn't you want to take care of one of the most precious gifts we could ever receive: the muscle part of the Lean Body Mass. If an athlete considered loaning you his or her body for a few weeks, how would you take care of such a high-performance body? Could you take care of your own body the same way?

What potential does your body have? The one that doesn't look or perform the way you want it to. It is interesting to think how those courageous individuals, who are handicapped, explore the limits of what they have. These people would see you as having unlimited potential. What would this person do with your body, the one that you complain about? If the athlete could take your body and maximize it, and someone who is physically limited could take it and gladly develop its potential, what about you? Are you wasting the opportunity or uncovering the potential?

Our muscle is willing and ready to perform completely. We are only required to feed it properly and exercise
it properly for its restoration. If we take care of the
muscle we have left, the other 30 to 70 per cent of
muscle that is not functioning because of inactivity will
return.

This background of the food and training balance
develops an appreciation that training programs and
food programs do work. The next step is to create a
vision of what you want for your future body. Think about
the rate of change you desire, and review the activities
you want to participate in, that will result in fat loss and
muscle gain.

How Good Will I Look and How Fast Can I Get There?

After a few years of working with people to change
body composition through food and training, I scheduled
my most challenging consultation. This person had completed college, raised a family, was successful in her
profession and was not at all pleased with her body. The
results of her body composition evaluation were disap-
pointing; yet they created a great motivation to change.

I knew this would be a major test for me. She had a
very demanding schedule, overweight parents and rela-
tives, had never been slender, or in shape and active ath-
letically. So therefore, she had no indication that improving her body was possible. I knew that many people
would benefit from her example if we could develop a
strategy to change her body.

Our conversation was brilliant! She understood completely that her body composition changes would
depend upon her own food and training program, and it

would take many months, if not a few years, for her to attain her goal. This was the first time I had witnessed anyone grasp the concept of long-term change in muscle and fat, and her own responsibility in the process. Basking in the fact that I had finally put together the perfect consultation, I asked: "Before we design your training program, is there anything else?"

"Just one more thing," she commented. "How good will I look, and how fast can I get there? My class reunion is next month!"

It's always amazing, and sometimes not obvious, to those of us in health care that after our absolute "best and most logical" consultations, which should lead people to the undeniable conclusion that improvement takes time, the reality is--emotion wins!

"How good will I look and how fast can I get there?" is, a very valid question. How you look now depends on the amount of your Lean Body Mass and position of your fat, which are the result of your food and training program up to this point. How you will look and how fast you will get there also depends on the amount of your Lean Body Mass, the position of your fat, *and* your food and training program from now on.

Creating a Vison

A major clue for developing a vision of how you want to look was expressed very well by the question of an astute observer:

"Why is it that we spend so much time on the front of us, when what we all notice about each other is the back of us?"

Start with a clear vision of how you want your body to look and perform. Include more than shape in your vision. Consider posture, movement, how your clothes fit, your body's contour, energy level and performance.

To begin your vision, consider the amount of lean mass you have at present, the level of activity you are currently engaged in, and the level of activity you are willing to undertake. The amount of muscle and how it is distributed on your body determines shape, performance level, and how fast you burn the stored fat calories.

Developing a vision requires thought, and moving toward that vision requires action. What would it be like to have a vision that in five years your body would be better than it has ever been, regardless of age? Can you imagine starting and continuing a program of weight and shape improvement for no other reason than you have created a vision, and that's the way it will be? Moving toward your vision demonstrates that you like yourself enough to improve. In addition, this process might increase the number of quality years you have to enjoy your family and friends.

Vision: Adding Muscle and Losing Fat

Initially, adding muscle means increasing the density or compactness of the muscle, *not the size*. As muscle becomes more toned, it becomes more dense and more metabolically active. This means it burns more fat calories. As the muscle increases in tone, there is less tendency for sagging tissue. Most women are reluctant to include adding lean mass as part of their goal or vision, until they learn that additional muscle tissue, without the fat, gives contour to their bodies; and that the more trained the muscle is, the more compact or small it becomes, and the more calories it uses per day.

Losing fat from the body has distinct rules, and a certain appearance, at various stages. The longer fat is on our body, the more dense it becomes. During the beginning stages of fat loss, there is less change in body size. Initially, as fat is lost, it becomes less dense, occupies the same space, then slowly begins to disappear, provided the improvement program continues. A body composition evaluation is the way to confirm fat loss even when there appears to be no change in size.

The direction of fat loss proceeds from the head downward. The head and neck area show the initial reduction of fat, then the shoulders, chest, ribs. Unfortunately, while we would like the lower areas to be first, fat loss is slower from the waist, hips and thighs.

How Fast I Can Change: Adding Lean

We all want to know our individual time frame, or rate of change, for adding lean and losing fat. Our best rate of improvement happens when food and training are balanced to our Lean Body Mass. Training is the activity responsible for creating Lean Body Mass and decreasing body fat. Once we understand how lean mass can be lost and gained, it is possible to begin controlling body fat.

Many people perform the right activities to add Lean Body Mass and don't see results, because they have disregarded or forgotten what causes muscle loss. My concern with loss of lean mass stems from the fact that with our activity level, values and awareness, or lack of awareness, of food, the loss of muscle portion of the Lean Body Mass is more common than we believe.

Recent studies have indicated that loss of muscle tissue is not confined to the muscles of our arms, legs, shoulders and back, even heart muscle can be lost. A recent article stated:

"A significant reduction in heart mass can occur within six weeks after overweight people start eating less. This is true even on a moderate diet of 1200 to 1500 calories per day. The more severe the diet, the greater the loss of heart mass possible." (Insight, January 18, 1988)

Training and eating properly could allow an increase in Lean Body Mass, of one or two pounds, every month. This rapid change happens with people who have lost lean mass, and are returning to their previous amount of muscle. As your lean mass approaches your genetic potential, the rate at which you progress decreases. It is possible, through a food and training program, to increase your lean mass past its genetic potential, depending on the intensity and type of training program you choose.

Maintaining the amount of Lean Body Mass you have is a desirable goal. When you are maintaining muscle mass, you are also preventing a loss of muscle, which is the most common problem in our society. Adding one pound of muscle mass to your body can accelerate the rate at which you lose body fat, provided you consume the same amount of food.

As muscle tissue becomes less active, it becomes less compact. Muscle that is not compact or completely toned occupies more space. It is more fluffy than highly active, performance muscles. As a person begins to train and condition the muscle, there is an increase in muscle density and a decrease in the muscle size. This is due to the loss of fat between the muscle fibers. Therefore, it is quite possible to be stronger and improve muscle shape without increasing muscle size.

What About Age?

The all-time great baseball player Sachel Paige said: "How old would you be if you didn't know how old you were?" What is your definition of age? For some, it is the number of years since birth. We all carry our opinions of what should happen at ages 40, 50, 60, 70 etc. The natural law is that your muscles don't know how old you are. Unfortunately, you know; therefore you establish certain limits on your muscles, according to your beliefs.

Recent evidence shows that elderly people can reap the same benefits from weight training as younger people. In a recent article, William J. Evans, Chief of the Physiology Lab at Tuft University's Research Center on Aging, studied twelve males, ages 60 to 72. In a twelve week period, they increased their ability to lift weights with their legs from 44 pounds to 85 pounds. Many increased their leg muscle size, some as much as 15%. The belief that older people generally cannot increase muscle size or strength is unfounded. Evans stated:

> "A high number of the elderly are profoundly weak, but expectations of what they can do should be raised, because they can respond well if asked to do a lot". Even people in their 80s and 90s can participate in weight training, according to Evans. He feels that the number of falls and injuries experienced by the elderly could be significantly reduced, if they strengthened muscle and connective tissue. Also stress response could be improved, since muscle mass contains protein that counteracts stress. (Insight, May 2, 1988)

You may draw your own conclusions regarding your age and future. However, we are all future senior citizens, and our energy level, performance and health are intimately connected with the muscle of our Lean Body Mass. If you are still undecided about training, there is one comment your LBM would make if it could speak:

"You are too old not to train!"

Fat Loss

How fast you can use stored body fat depends upon the amount of time you spend at your optimum, fat loss, Training Heart Rate, the amount of Lean Body Mass you have, and how you train each week.

One pound of fat contains approximately 3600 calories. Assuming you are eating the correct percentages of proteins, fats and carbohydrates, a deficiency of 500 calories per day would result, mathematically speaking, in one pound of fat loss every seven days. We can safely assume at least half of the calories used during exercise are from fat, if we are training and using food properly. Body composition results indicate that for most of us one pound of fat loss every two weeks is more realistic.

Wonder diets that claim five to ten pounds of weight loss per week don't explain that the weight loss is made up of water, muscle and a small percentage of fat. For the ten pound loss to be composed of all stored body fat, a person would have to use an extra 36,000 calories in one week, or the same amount of energy required to run one and one-half marathons per day, for seven days.

Before you go into deep despair, read further. There have been many unrealistic stories and myths about fat loss. It is time for the truth. *Fat loss takes time*. Regardless of what you read or hear about rapid fat loss, there are natural laws that are absolutely true, and are not influenced by what we believe. One such law is: We must expend 3,600 extra calories to lose one pound of fat.

The human trait is to believe that our five pound weight loss in two days is definitely all fat. Adding five pounds of "scale weight" over the weekend would mean eating and storing 18,000 *extra* calories as body fat.

It is more likely that the sudden increase in scale weight is a change in the amount of water our body contains. Our body stores water in varying amounts; so don't be alarmed at sudden changes in scale weight. These are words to live by when using your scale to determine if your weekend was a success:

"Scales rarely tell the whole truth!"

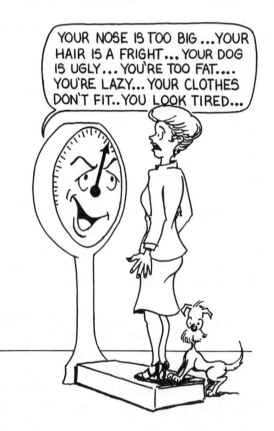

Sudden increases or decreases in scale weight are water fluctuations. It may take months before you completely stop worrying about a two to three pound change in body water, which is much less of a problem as you become more lean and more trained.

Changing Your Body: It Takes Time

When one compares the time it takes to become thin to the time it takes to become lean, thin wins every time. Getting thin requires no activity, very little food, and it happens almost automatically. Being thin, meaning small in size, is generally characterized by a low Lean Body Mass, poor muscle tone and a high percentage of fat. Thin people usually have a low energy level, tire easily and add pounds to their body with very little food.

Many people choose thin rather than lean because thin is faster and easier. They do not want weight loss to take a long time. This is another reminder of the natural law: *It takes time*; and the human trait: *I want it now*!

People's time perspective is interesting. We will spend ten years using plans that don't improve our body or change it for the worse; and, yet, we find it hard to consider spending ten years changing for the better. When we finally decide to improve, the general attitude is: How fast can we get there?

Occasionally we actually become discouraged when we learn how long it would take to accomplish weight and shape goals. There are some absolute laws that cannot be changed with man-made gimmicks, fad diets, pills and shortcuts. It is far more important to realize that our body is a perfect representation of our current food and training program.

Changing Your Body: What Happens

Even though we have heard that it takes years to accumulate fat and develop a shape we don't like, it seems that one day we look in the mirror and we are suddenly different. We did not change overnight; yet it seems as if our body got out of shape while we were not paying attention.

If the body had the ability to hook up to a computer, the printout would have a mark at each loss of lean mass, or gain in body fat, which would say: illness, special diet, inactive period, too busy to eat, and so on. When we become aware of weight control, body shape, who looks good and who doesn't, we want improvement fast! The secret to rapid improvement is: If you are impatient about changing your body, then be impatient about monitoring your body composition!

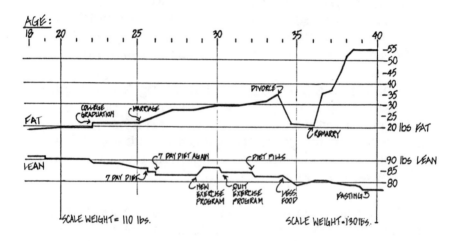

Figure 21 - How the body changes over time

What's Possible: Your Body's Rate of Improvement

Most of us would like major improvements in our weight and shape by the weekend. Let's look at an example of what the body can do when we provide the right environment, in terms of a proper food and training program. Keep in mind that the following example is what we call being realistic.

In this example the client actually considered time, cooking, shopping, interest, intensity, family, vacations and making it fun. Her first body composition evaluation was:

Weight	135 pounds
Lean Body Mass	80 pounds
Fat	55 pounds

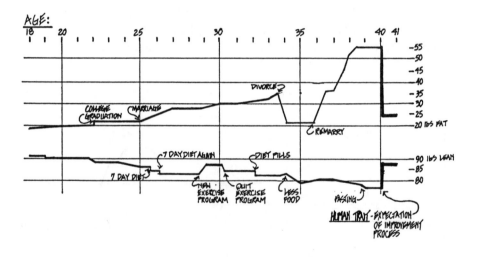

Figure 22 - Our Initial Expectation of the Improvement Process

Her Initial Expectations: Initialially, her goal was to lose 30 pounds in six weeks (five per week) and maintain this weight loss. 30 pounds is not realistic, and the concern with rapid weight loss is that 30 pounds in six weeks consists of eight to fifteen pounds of muscle, ten to fifteen pounds of water, and five to seven pounds of fat. At eighty pounds of lean mass, (about thirty pounds of muscle), this individual can not afford to lose even one pound of muscle mass!

Her Realistic Program: An active lifestyle, with minimum time for training and many meals away from home, requires balancing food to her Lean Body Mass. I suggested a fat loss rate of approximately one pound per month, and the more important change of an increase in muscle mass, with the following benefits:

1. Being able to eat more calories.
2. Having more energy at the end of the day.
3. Increasing muscle mass capacity to burn more fat.

The results could be accomplished in one year, more realistically in two, depending upon her training schedule. Certainly they are achievable in three or four years.

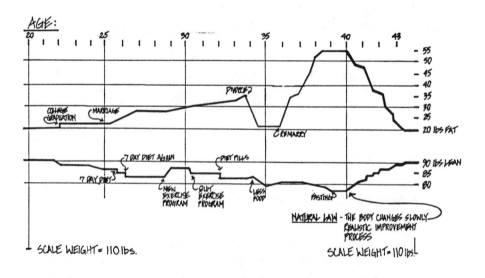

Figure 23 - A Realistic Program

Figure 24 - A Realistic Program: Rate of Change

	CURRENT	16th MONTH	38th MONTH
Weight	135 pounds	122 pounds	110 pounds
Lean	80 pounds	85 pounds	90 pounds
Muscle Portion of Lean Mass	25 lbs	+5 lbs muscle (30 lbs total)	+10 lbs muscle (35 lbs total)
Fat	55 lbs	-18 lbs fat (37 lbs left)	-25 lbs fat (20 lbs left)
% Lean - % Fat	60% - 40%	70% - 30%	82% - 18%

Discussion of Figure 23 and 24: At the 16 month point, notice that a five pound increase in muscle is a 20% increase in the power and energy of her body, even if nothing else changes. The added bonus of reducing 55 pounds of fat to 37 pounds (a decrease of 18%) makes her 20% increase in muscle power go even further.

What is it worth in your life to have 20% more energy, and decrease the excess fat you carry by 18%? What if this change took 24 months? Would it still be worth it? You are going to be two years older anyway.

Look at the change that has occurred by the 38th month: another five pounds increase in lean mass and a seventeen pound decrease in fat. What would it be like if you were four years older, and had 30% more energy and a 20%-50% decrease in the extra fat you carry with you throughout the day? The rewards for this woman were more than physical; she learned to control weight and shape, how to recover from a setback and how to improve in spite of age and a busy schedule.

Even if it takes two, three or four years to reach your goals, isn't it exciting to get better as you get older? These results are not available in a two or four week program, or even in a $2,500 one-week fat farm program.

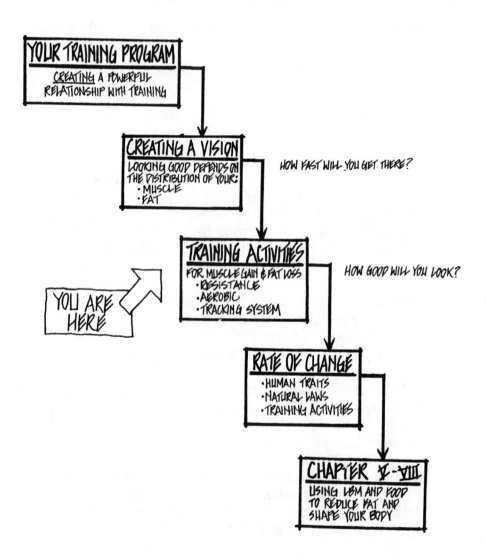

Activities that Change Lean Mass and Body Fat

Perhaps it would be useful to consider a new approach to training. If training were thought of as a tool we used to get a specific result, we would focus on the result we wanted and use the activity as a means of achieving it. Some training activities create muscle; others cause fat loss. The question to ask yourself is: If I participate in this training activity, what can I expect?

Regardless of our reasons and our level of training, we all have the same questions and concerns:

● Is our program working?

● Is it working fast enough?

● Will it hurt?

There are many myths and misconceptions about training and rate of change. There are also expectations we have, and time schedules to work around. How can we find or create the best program for the fastest results? While there is not one answer that will make our program easy, there are many truths that will keep us from wasting time and effort on ineffective training programs. This chapter is to help us build a base, and establish our own training program. The two major categories for training are resistance and aerobic.

Gaining or Maintaining Muscle Mass

It is possible, to see the best trainers following the best training program, with absolutely no increase in muscle mass. An important key to using an activity to gain muscle is to learn what might prevent the program from working. The missing ingredient is the balancing of food with training, for that particular individual. Once the proper food program has been established, there are three specific requirements for adding muscle:

1. It is essential to have a program that changes every four to eight weeks, because the body adapts rapidly to any activity or exercise. If you continually provide the body with new stimulation by varying your training, the body will respond by adding or developing the muscle part of your Lean Body Mass.

2. An equally important factor in adding muscle is the manner in which the exercise is performed. This is another way of saying that proper form, or how you do a particular exercise, is critical to your success.

3. With resistance training, the presence of a coach or trainer will be an important part of your support team. You will want to work with a coach who has a successful personal program, as well as success with people you can talk to about their progress.

The desire to gain muscle or lose fat is more than matched with "miracle" drugs, products and systems to create great results overnight. Inevitably, when talking about gaining Lean Body Mass, the issue of using steroids for rapid muscle gain is discussed. Current literature, and especially magazines such as *Muscle and Fitness*, covers this subject very well, and quite thoroughly. The only comment I would add is this: We are, as a culture, impatient and want instant results and gratification in all areas. Using steroids to increase muscle or surgery to remove fat means always having to depend on an outside source or person to have body you want. Any attempt to trick the body is very expensive, in terms of time, emotion and money.

It is important to have a yardstick, or gauge, we can use to measure any new or different program. If a program is one that you can only use for a short time, because long-term use will result in illness, degeneration of your lean mass, or even "death", then why do it at all? Although the word death seems fairly harsh in this context, it may stimulate you to look objectively at some of the fad programs and diets which promise rapid weight change in a short time. A few months to a year on one of these programs would result in extreme degeneration of Lean Body Mass.

The specific activities that work for increasing Lean Body Mass are termed resistance training. The particular systems used are free weights, exercise machines such as Nautilus, Universal gym equipment and any exercise equipment, that allows you to increase the amount of tension or weight as your body adapts to the activity. For exercises and training, I refer you to any number of books on the subject, and also to the vast number of magazines currently available on every sport, activity and training that we know of.

The literature will increase your interest and awareness to a point where, ultimately, it will be necessary to work with a coach or trainer for maximum results. It is not the exercise equipment that creates the body you want; it is how the equipment is used. We cannot have the body we want without adequate Lean Body Mass, and we cannot see the body we have created if it is hiding beneath fat.

Losing Fat

Fat loss can be accomplished with almost any activity that will sustain a certain training heart rate for 30 to 90 minutes. Rather than select an activity you may not like, I suggest learning the basics of fat loss, and then you can adapt almost any of your favorite activities to your program. If you have no favorite activities, once you understand the principles of fat loss, you may begin a training program on the basis of which activity has the least number of objections. Some of the better activities for fat loss are: walking, slow jogging, biking (mobile or stationary), cross-country skiing or cross-country skiing machines, rowing machines, swimming, and any activity that allows you to be in control of the consistent training heart rate.

Aerobic dance activities can result in fat loss, if one eats properly and monitors her or his heart rate. One of the many advantages of aerobic classes is that they inspire participation. Unfortunately, unless the person is eating extremely well, we see very little change in fat loss, or muscle gain, with aerobic dance activities. Aerobic dance instructors, now assist participants in managing their Training Heart Rate throughout the exercise session. A balanced eating plan and body composition evaluations to monitor results, might also motivate students to participate in the class.

Keep these points in mind:

- Participants can become involved in the excitement of the class causing their heart rates to go much too high for fat loss.

- Attending class four or more times per week is necessary to accomplish a change.

- The body adapts to any activity. What works for participants at week 10 may not work at week 20.

Body composition evaluations at the advised two to four week intervals help to determine if additional training is necessary to accomplish your goals.

Monitoring Systems

As we have mentioned throughout these chapters, the body composition evaluation is not only a tremendous incentive to keep you on track with your food and training, but it is also an indicator of how your Lean Body Mass is responding to various programs and situations.

Illness can cause a rapid reduction in Lean Body Mass, as can fasting and diets. It seems as though Lean Body Mass can decrease faster than fat can increase. Teaching your body to gain lean mass and lose fat is a skill; and depending on the time you have been inactive, your body needs to learn how to change. The body does not build muscle or use fat because we want it to happen.

Often a person will read a book, begin to exercise and expect the lean mass to increase, with a decrease in fat, within a week. The body has its own reality and proceeds at the pace that it perceives as normal within each person's food and training program. The purpose of monitoring is to prevent the loss of lean mass, or the increase of fat, from going unnoticed, and to keep us focused on a training and food program that works.

What Gauge or Monitor can be Used?

When training, our body uses two types of fuel: fat and carbohydrates. What's needed is a gauge or indicator to tell us the kind of fuel we are using, and what is happening with our body composition. Fortunately, we have two gauges designed to give us this information: a body composition evaluation and our Training Heart Rate.

The body composition evaluation can be the basic indicator system of resistance training. Although this system is outside the body, it tells you how you have done with your food and training program during the last two to four weeks. It will also inform you whether you need to consume more or less proteins, fats or carbohydrates.

Your Training Heart Rate is the basic indicator system of aerobic training. This system is inside the body, and tells you from moment to moment if you are burning carbohydrates or fat for fuel. What more could you ask?

Training Heart Rate

Just as monitoring the amount of lean mass can be an indicator of how well your program is working, the body has a built-in monitor to provide you constant feedback about your most efficient rate of fat loss. This monitoring system is called your Training Heart Rate (THR). It tells you how many calories you are using, and whether those calories are from stored body fat or stored carbohydrates.

Losing fat efficiently depends on the "right" THR, and not how fast or how far you run. Your best Training Heart Rate for fat loss is a simple calculation (Figure 25, p. 133). Your best fat loss heart rate will be unique to you. It will also change as you improve. When you have been inactive, it is important to begin at a lower heart rate to give your body an opportunity to learn a new skill called "fat loss."

Taking Your Six Second Pulse

1. Find your pulse by placing your forefinger and index finger on either the inside of your wrist or the side of your throat just under the jaw.

2. Count the number of beats in a six second amount of time

3. Multiply the number of beats in six seconds by 10 for your pulse per minute.

If your pulse rate is between numbers at the six second mark, count a halfbeat. Example: If your pulse rate is between eight and nine, use 8.5 in your calculations, which would give you a pulse rate of 85 beats per minute.

Use the six second pulse method to calculate both your resting and Training Heart Rate.

Figure 25 - Training Heart Rate (THR)

EXPLANATION	EXAMPLE	FORMULA
1. Start with the number220	220	220
2. Subtract your age	<u>-45</u> (example)	<u>-</u>___ (your age)
Your theoretical maximum heart rate/minute	175	
3. Subtract your resting heart rate	<u>-75</u> (example)	<u>-</u>___ (resting)
4. If you are just beginning, Multiply by 45% or 50%	<u>x0.45</u>	<u>x</u>___
5. Addyour resting heart rate	<u>+75</u> (example)	<u>+</u>___ (resting)
Your THR/minute	**120**	

Figure 26 - The Target Zone for Your THR

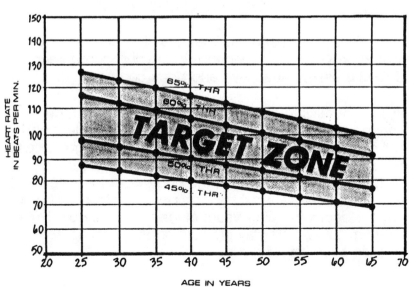

TARGET ZONE HEART RATES

How to Start

If you have been inactive for a period of time, or have been involved in some form of exercise for years without the results you want, consider **re**-starting your training program.

1. Begin by walking. Use this activity to learn about and experience your Training Heart Rate (THR). An activity you prefer can be substituted for walking.

2. At first, walk ten minutes each day or twice a day as your time permits. Add five to ten minutes each week until you reach 30 to 60 minutes a day. How long and how often depends upon your goals.

3. Your individual THR is a percentage of your theoretical maximum rate. Initially, use 45% to 50% for two weeks, then increase 5% every two weeks until you reach 65%. Stay at this percentage for six to twelve months.

4. Give your body time to adapt. Encourage yourself to be patient, and avoid increasing too rapidly.

5. Keep a journal of your activity. The consistency of your improvement will depend upon your record keeping of food, training, heart rate and body composition.

Do not fall into the trap of thinking that you know what heart rate is best for your fat loss. It is a clear and well-documented fact that your heart knows a great deal more about your best rate of fat loss training than your mind. To burn fat efficiently, the body must train slowly at its fat-loss heart rate over a long period of time. Long, if you are beginning after years of inactivity, may be five to fifteen minutes, and may increase to as much as an hour or more over many weeks.

You may find it reassuring to know that the Training Heart Rate is quite low for fat loss. This means you can lose fat walking at a moderate pace. If you are having a difficult time breathing during activity, you are overdoing it. Gradually work up to a time in minutes which uses up the number of calories you chose for that day or session.

Many people feel they have not exercised hard enough when training at their fat burning heart rate. Fat loss is a function of your heart rate, not your mind and what you think. When we are training at too high a heart rate, oxygen is not as abundant in the muscle cells. Fat loss is not as efficient under these conditions. Our first clue that the heart rate is too high is that we are breathing too hard to carry on a conversation.

The next question is always, "How long should I train at my THR and how many times per week?" It has been determined that while your muscles use both fat and carbohydrates, and even some protein during activity, the muscles initially use 75% to 80% carbohydrates during the first 15 minutes of activity. This approaches 50% carbohydrates and 50% fat during the first 30 to 40 minutes. At the one-hour point, it is possible to be using 75% of the calories in fat. From this data, we could assume that one hour or more at our fat loss heart rate is better. Initially, the untrained person can accomplish significant results with shorter periods of time in activity.

As our body composition improves and the body becomes more efficient, it may be necessary to increase time spent and frequency per week to accomplish the desired results. There are no hard and fast rules regarding your body and your results. During the initial stages, find out what works for you in terms of time and days per week, and keep a journal of your activity and your body composition results. The body is very efficient and adapts to whatever we do. What works for you at the six week period will not work at week twelve. That means you must adjust your Training Heart Rate, time and frequency of activity in order to continue your improvement.

Most literature will suggest a frequency of three times a week for your training or activity. It is reported in some journals that three times per week will keep you right where you are today, and four to five times a week is necessary for you to improve. I have seen this statement proven and disproven. You must find out what works best for your body and for your schedule.

Designing Your Training Plan

The next step is to design a program based on your goals, and then have the training create your body. Because most of us have very little time in our busy day to train. Your first bit of homework in designing your training program is to create your weekly schedule in advance, and schedule one-hour of training each day of the week. Can you imagine, after establishing that there is no available time, someone asks you to set aside or create an additional hour per day for training? People are initially confused and ask questions like: "Why every day? Isn't three times a week enough?" "I don't have five minutes a day; how can I find time for one hour a day?"

It is a human tendency to believe something about the future, and then justify the belief as though it were already fact. There are no future facts. My request is for you to look at your schedule ahead of time, and create 60 minutes per day for training. Make this a challenge, to see if you can create training time within a week that you believe is already filled.

The second part of your homework is as follows: Make a list, using your creativity, of the reasons you might have for training that are more inspirational, and have a higher purpose than "Training is an inconvenience in my busy schedule." Example are: involving an out-of-shape friend, in your exercise program; spending one hour walking and communicating, while sharing time and activity with your spouse or other family members; listening to inspirational tapes in the morning as you train -- before school, work or before the family wakes up; being an example physically for your family; being healthy enough to actively participate in family sports with your children and grandchildren, and so on.

The more reasons you write down, the more your initial reasons for not training, such as busy schedule and inconvenience, become smaller and less significant. Your reasons become a source of motivation and inspiration, which have a positive influence on the people around you. Let's have our approach to our bodies, succeed in a way that is not only a model for family and friends, but also a demonstration that we are in control of our weight, shape and performance at any age.

Wrapping Up

We can't simply talk and design training programs. Eventually, we actually have to go to the track or to the gym, start riding the bike, or go to the aerobics class and perform. Our performance literally shouts who we are. The next time you walk into an exercise class or gym, watch the people for a while and answer these questions. Who is alive? Who is maximizing his or her potential? Who is getting the most out of class? Which of these people would I want to be?

Training and improving your body is really a gift that you give to yourself. You and I both know it is much easier to give a gift to someone you like, rather than to someone you don't like. It is time to consider a relationship with a part of your body that you already like and already have, your Lean Body Mass. It is easier to like yourself when you can recognize and appreciate the alive part of you - the part that is *really* you.

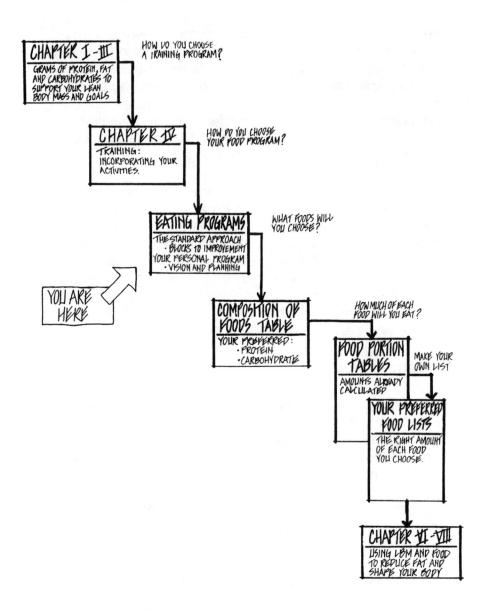

CHAPTER 5

Designing Your Food Program

"To the blind, all things are sudden."
Old Russian Saying

Overview

According to our beliefs, all fat loss should be sudden. According to our body, fat is accumulated slowly and lost slowly. This is one of the natural laws. While we know this is true, when it comes to our own rate of fat loss, we don't believe it! Our minds still believe the fat should go suddenly!

We could say that a short attention span and strong beliefs are definite characteristics of our minds. Some of the strongest beliefs we have are about our food. We have also developed habits which support our beliefs, even when they do not work for us. Strong beliefs can blind us to possibilities.

Let's imagine that you have just purchased the most expensive, high performance automobile available, and have been using a low quality fuel which was mistakenly placed in the gas station's extra high performance fuel pump. The car would perform poorly. You would believe the car was a lemon. The dealer would believe you were making it up. The mechanic would use electronic testers to tune the engine, and double and triple check all mechanisms on this elaborate automobile, only to find all systems working perfectly.

The car manufacturer would believe that everyone was wrong, and the net overall result would be the car continuing to run poorly. After months of confrontation-- your opinions about the dealership and the dealership's opinions about you, the opinions of multiple experts, more tests--you might get very lucky and someone might determine . . . it's the fuel!

Similarly, our beliefs and opinions about our bodies prevent us from seeing possibilities. In a not-too-imaginary situation, it is possible that, after years of treating the symptoms of weight, shape and other ailments we believe mysteriously happen to us, we may find that in reality . . . it's the fuel!

Food Programs: The Hidden Problem

Designing our own food program can be far more effective than using standard eating plans. We ordinarily do not consider how we are eating as the problem, because it is normal, average and/or what we have always done. Even diets become "normal" after a time, because we have always been on a diet of some type. We never look at our weight, excess fat, or being out of shape as the result or symptom of a problem. Instead, we see the condition that we don't like as the problem itself, and want this situation corrected. We look for answers and solutions about what programs to follow, what pills to take, what gimmicks to use and what new information to learn. Could the way we have been eating and dieting be the cause of the problem?

The real issue is that we never question our usual patterns, because we are too busy looking for the next new program to bring about a quick change. If we examine the *reasons* or possible causes for our symptoms, such as fat and being out of shape, then "what to do about them and how to prevent them" is an entirely different issue.

Whenever we read a book about food, relative to weight loss, our bodies or cooking, we always look for what to eat. An emphasis on what foods to eat does not create winning in the weight loss game. Evidence clearly demonstrates that telling people what to eat doesn't work. It is far more effective to become aware of the effect food has on our own body, before making choices about "what to eat."

Looking at food as both the cause and the cure of our weight and shape problems, puts us in the position of control in selecting our foods. Creating a strong and effective eating program requires being aware of barriers such as; the emotional effect of eating programs, what we want physically and where we look for answers, and how we usually eat.

The Emotional Effect

What we go through emotionally, regarding food, is common, and totally unnecessary. We eat the way we always have, or subscribe to various diet programs; and then become emotional, or feel guilty, as if we personally were wrong about our bodies not responding to these programs. We forget, or have never learned, that our standard eating approach and the majority of food programs on the market today are not designed for long-term success. The more we stay on these programs, or eat in a way that does not balance the Lean Body Mass, the more out of shape and discouraged we get.

Most conversations concerning weight, shape or eating, are opinions and concerns about what we read and hear from the various experts, and programs. The information and the programs appear to work initially. Ultimately, however, they stop working and we fail to reach our desired results. An element of guilt is always present regarding what we couldn't do, how there was not enough time, and how we should have eaten better. Sometimes we become discouraged when we realize it has been years since we have seen any type of improvement. We have tried everything, struggled; and we are now 20 pounds heavier. In the final stages of the battle, we deny the extra pounds, or just accept "the way it is" with excuses of genetics, nothing works anyway, and we just don't have enough time.

What We Want and Where We Look for Anwsers

What we want and expect for our body from our food program is fascinating: more weight loss, a better shape and a higher energy level as soon as possible, and with very little inconvenience. Where we look for improvement, and how we monitor our progress, is even more fascinating. For our weight, we consult the bathroom scale, which knows nothing about body composition. For our shape, we consult the most available mirror, or our clothing. Mirrors, we learn, withhold the real truth from us for years; and one day when the mirror is in a bad mood, it reveals all. For our energy level, we consult our mind.

Using the mirror, the scale and our own thoughts for information creates standard and predictable actions: We eat less, try diet plans, take vitamins, work with our mind to visualize ourselves full of energy and in great shape. In reality, our weight, shape, energy level and performance are the result of our Lean Body Mass and fat.

Rather than relying on the bathroom scale, mirror or our mind, we can find accurate and personal information by looking at the following:

- Our body composition, the proportion of Lean Body Mass and fat.

- Our weight in terms of Lean Body Mass.

- Our shape in terms of our body's proportion of Lean Body Mass and fat.

- Our body tone--firm or soft muscle.

How We Usually Eat

We usually eat according to various habits that we have acquired over the years, and according to what we like, regardless of its effect on our bodies. We are easily influenced when it comes to food. What we think, hear and see, relative to pictures of food, quick weight-loss claims, fad diets and even smells, can influence not only what, but how much and when we eat. The standard approach is to eat the food, and then hope the result will not be very bad.

When we begin to suspect that food is a part of our problem, we take one or more of the following steps:

1. We eat whatever food is available first, and ask questions later.

2. We know our food program isn't the best, so we take vitamins.

3. We decide it is the quantity of food, and begin our version of eating less, moderately interspersed with binges as a reward for eating less.

4. We use organized systems, such as fad diet plans, which have short-term benefits.

5. We read, become experts, and ask other "experts" what they do with different weight/shape programs.

It should be obvious by this point that the random approach doesn't work, and yet it is very common. Let's begin building an approach that will work for you, one that is totally personalized and designed to allow optimum improvement in your weight, shape and performance *indefinitely*.

The Tools for an Effective Food Program?

Food and training programs always give us a result. In order to obtain the result we want, food must be eaten in a way that supports our body. The tools you need to begin are different from the standard, and rigid food plans. The tools are actually the *basic requirements* necessary to create the success you want from your food and training programs. These requirements are:

- **Vision**. A vision of where your body will be. This, of course, will include your goals for weight, shape and performance.

- **Context**. A context or whole picture of your improvement, including: training, your on-going food program, a timetable for your improvement, your schedule and your support system.

- **Information**. This includes LBM and your food and training requirements, such as LBM amount and your personal food and training preferences.

- **Planning**. With the information available, you can chose and create a food plan and a schedule that will work in all situations, for life.

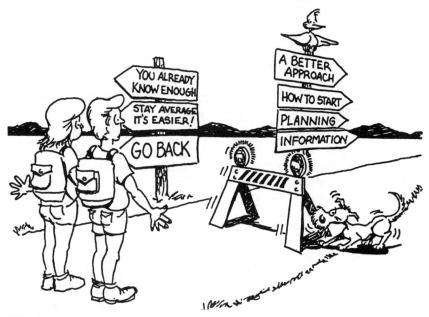

Vision

Start your vision by picturing the alive part of you, the Lean Body Mass, arranged the way you want it to be, with as little or as much fat as you choose. Your vision totally disregards history, is not based on time (weeks or months), and is a pure statement of what you want for your body, in terms of Lean Body Mass, fat, energy level, weight and shape. After establishing your vision, you can begin to work with goals, objectives and time periods.

Context

Our standard thinking about food rarely has positive results. Attempting to improve by eating first, and hoping the results will be what we want, not only doesn't work; it is backwards. If you were to start at the end of this sentence and read the words backwards, one at a time, it would be confusing to your mind. What reading backwards does to your mind, eating randomly does to your body: confusion! Your body is not confused by a balanced of protein, fat and carbohydrates, eaten in a way that matches your Lean Body Mass.

Understanding the total picture of food, from Lean Body Mass to actually preparing and eating the food, is similar to taking a class at school. When it comes to completing school work, a few students can be given assignments or details, and they actually construct their own context or overview. Most of us, however, need an overview first; and then we can make sense of the details and daily assignments. We have learned that telling people exactly what foods to eat is the same as giving them details. An overview is needed to put food in perspective.

All eating is for life. Just because we eat every day, food is available, and we are "informed dieters" does not mean that we know what is best for our LBM. Also, it doesn't mean we can make sense of all the opinions and advice about the food we are exposed to every day. Creating a context for your improvement requires that you step back for a time and look at the complete picture of food, relative to your body composition and the information you have learned to this point.

Information

Data gathering is absolutely vital to create a context and perspective for your individual food program. An accurate and effective method of data gathering is to:

1. Eat according to your percentage plan for protein and carbohydrate.

2. Record your food and training accurately in a journal.

3. Use your body composition evaluation at two-week intervals to indicate how you have done, and to establish your next "two-week experiment" and data-gathering session.

Your personal data, based on your own experience, is effective, tells you exactly what is happening with your body, and helps establish a plan for the next two to four week period. Using an outline allows you to establish a plan which is designed to match individual requirements. You will notice that every aspect of your food plan is influenced by your choices or your body in some way. While most food plans are standardized, we, as humans, are highly individualized. We all have different food preferences, ages, activity levels, training programs, and Lean Body Mass amounts, not to mention goals and various means of approaching this project. It is absolutely vital that a plan--your individual plan--is created.

Planning

Planning not only includes a perspective of food from Lean Body Mass to what you eat; it also includes a perspective of time, in terms of days, weeks, hours and years. It seems as though the issue of time is always at the center of our discussions about food, weight, training and shape. When people consider the time it will take to lose fat, train every day, shop and plan, they usually say things such as:

- The days and weeks go too fast.

- Exercise takes too much time.

- Getting back into shape takes to long.

- Getting out of shape happens overnight.

These four contrasting viewpoints on the same subject, time, should be enough to convince you that our perspective of time can be inaccurate, depends on our mood, and is not in harmony with how the body relates to time. The body has a more reliable concept of time than our "minds," when it comes to how fast we can lose fat, gain muscle, and reach our goals.

With planning, perhaps time is something we could be more "in control of" rather than be "controlled by." If we could be in control of time and food, it is possible that we would eliminate 90% of the complaints that dominate our daily conversations.

All people who have had extraordinary success in achieving the body composition they wanted have had these tools in their foundation. It seemed that, as they grasped the concept of vision, context, information and planning, their rate of progress accelerated. This is not a specific type of person, but rather someone who made a choice about no longer being satisfied with where his or her body is now, and where she or he is headed. Rather than wait until you achieve your ideal body, develop these tools now, ahead of time, and use them to create your body. These tools, are built into the design of each of us, and they appear when you interact with them.

Creating a Food Program

After many attempts at using various methods to improve weight, shape, energy and performance, we get to a point where we want results from our effort. We become very interested in the truth, in something that will work for life, rather than just for a few weeks. With a personalized food program based on Lean Body Mass, your improvement is inevitable.

Once you know your Lean Body Mass, and select your goal for body composition, how much you eat and what you choose to eat is automatic. There will be less pressure from the constant decisions, choices, and mental gymnastics we perform regarding our food programs.

How Much Food?

The charts and tables in Chapters one through three have been designed to take you from LBM to grams per meal. The next step is to make a list of the foods you like, and then determine how much of each preferred food you will need. In most cases, with the exception of high fat foods, the amount is more than we think. Food and diet plans always start by telling us which foods to eat. We read these food lists with the hope that what they tell us to eat will be something we like. A plan that works starts with your preferred foods and builds from there. Most of the foods you like can be part of your plan. This is not a program of eliminating foods; it is a plan to include your food in a way that supports you and your goals.

Because of the body composition evaluations and various tables, your food program choices can now be made with awareness. You will begin to learn which foods, and in what amount create the results you want for your body.

What to Eat

When someone asks me what to eat, I start with, "What do you like?" People review the Composition of Foods Table and select the foods they like. The Composition of Foods Table could be considered a food "dictionary." Reading through this dictionary not only helps us identify the foods we like, it also provides a breakdown of each food into its protein, fat and carbohydrate components.

You will notice that the table also gives the gram amounts for each food component. The food table is not just another interesting set of facts; it can be used to accelerate your rate of change by pointing out foods that, without your awareness, undermine progress.

The Composition of Foods Table

Before using the table we will alter the way in which foods are classified, by using a classification system that will make your choices easier, eliminate confusion, and help identify foods that stand in the way of your progress.

The purpose of food classification is to quickly and easily identify the foods that are high in fat, so we can avoid them; and the foods that are high in protein or high in carbohydrates, and low in fat, so we include them.

This is an example of how the new system works. We "know," because "everyone knows," that cheese and peanut butter are protein foods. The new system immediately labels both a high fat food. This does not mean you have to avoid or eliminate them from your diet, it means you now have to be responsible for the hundreds of extra fat grams that convert to fat on your body.

The following steps will introduce you to the Composition of Foods Table. (These are example foods chosen randomly from the table. See Appendix One for the complete table.)

Step 1: Read through the food table and identify all the foods you like, or are interested in, by placing a check mark next to the name.

EXAMPLE

Standard Portions
100 grams or 3 1/2 ounces

Food	Cal Gms	Pro Gms	Fat Gms	Carb Gms
- **Macaroni & Cheese**	215	8.4	11.1	20.1
- **Hamburger, cooked**	286	24.2	20.3	0.0

Step 2: Review the table again, with a red highlighter pen, and look at the column indicating grams of fat. Highlight any of your foods that have more than nine grams of fat in the 3 1/2 ounce (100 gram) portion.

EXAMPLE FOR HIGH FAT FOODS

Standard Portions
100 grams. or 3 1/2 ounces

	Food	Cal	Pro Gms	Fat Gms	Carb Gms
-	American Cheese	370	23.2	**30.0**	1.9
-	Chocolate Chip Cookies	471	5.4	**21.0**	69.7
-	Sunflower Seeds	560	24.0	**47.3**	19.9

Step 3: Review the table again, with a yellow highlighter pen, and look at the column indicating protein. Any protein food that has a "+" in the left hand margin is a complete protein with an acceptable amount of fat. Highlight your preferred protein foods that have 15 or more grams of protein in the 3 1/2 ounce portion. Place the yellow mark off to the left.

EXAMPLE FOR PROTEIN FOODS

Standard Portions
100 grams or 3 1/2 ounces

	Food	Cal	Pro Gms	Fat Gms	Carb Gms
+	Turkey, skinned, cooked	190	**31.5**	6.1	0.0
-	Peanut Butter	589	**25.2**	50.6	18.8
-	Ham, cooked	389	**16.9**	35.0	0.3

Step 4: Review the table for carbohydrates. These will be all your remaining checked foods. Use a blue highlighter to mark all of your remaining foods that have at least ten times more carbohydrate grams than fat grams. Any food that has a "*" in the left hand column is a carbohydrate with an acceptable amount of fat.

EXAMPLE FOR CARBOHYDRATE FOODS

Standard Portions
100 grams or 3 1/2 ounces

	Food	Cal	Pro Gms	Fat Gms	Carb Gms
*	Potato, baked	93	2.6	0.1	**21.1**
-	Potato Salad	145	3.0	9.2	**13.4**
*	Pasta, cooked	111	3.4	0.4	**23.0**

Step 5: Check the food table and boldly mark and identify any preferred or interesting foods that do not measure up to the ratio standard.

Ratio Standards: Protein

To be a protein, for our purposes, the food must have a protein-fat ratio of *at least* two protein to one fat, in grams. Five or more grams of protein to one fat gram is much better. If the protein is less than a five to one ratio, color over the yellow highlighter with the red highlighter pen. The higher fat, protein food will be easily identified because of the orange color.

Ratio Standards: Carbohydrates

The criteria for carbohydrates are similar. A ratio of ten carbohydrates to one fat is acceptable. If the carbohydrate is less than a ten to one ratio, color over the blue highlighter with the red highlighter pen. The higher fat, carbohydrate food will be easily identified because of the purple color.

EXAMPLE RATIO STANDARDS: PROTEIN

Standard Portions
100 grams or 3 1/2 ounces

	Food	Cal	Pro Gms	Fat Gms	Carb Gms
-	**2 : 1 Ratio** Ground Beef, lean, cooked	219	**27.4**	**11.3**	0.0
+/-	**5 : 1 Ratio** Chicken, skinned, roasted	183	**29.5**	**6.3**	0.0
+	**14 : 1 Ratio** 2% Lowfat Cottage Cheese	90	**14.0**	**1.0**	5.0

EXAMPLE RATIO STANDARDS: CARBOHYDRATE

Standard Portions
100 grams or 3 1/2 ounces

	Food	Cal	Pro Gms	Fat Gms	Carb Gms
*/-	**5 : 1 Ratio** Pizza, w/cheese, frozen	245	9.5	**7.1**	**35.4**
*	**12 : 1 Ratio** Bread, enriched, white	275	9.0	**4.0**	**50.0**
*	**233 : 1 Ratio** Rice, enriched, cooked	106	2.1	**0.1**	**23.3**

FOOD IDENTIFICATION SUMMARY

FOOD:	COLOR:
High Fat	Red
Protein	Yellow
Carbohydrate	Blue
Protein with higher fat	Orange
Carbohydrate with higher fat	Purple

The excessive fat in the American diet can be easily identified using this classification. You now can determine which foods fit into your goals.

The Foods You Like -- How Much?

Identify the foods you like and begin by recording your favorite carbohydrates in the Preferred Food List (Figure 27, p. 155). The amount of each food along with the fat content is listed in the Food Portion Table (Figure 28, p. 156-57). Circle the grams of carbohydrate you need per meal and match this with a food you like. A specific example of using the Food Portion Table is given on page 160 (Figure 31). Follow this example closely. The exercise will serve you well with all carbohydrate foods.

Fill in the Preferred Food List for Protein (Figure 29, page 158), and use the Food Portion Table for Protein, (Figure 30, page 159) to learn the amount you need and fat content of each food. Use the example on page 161 (Figure 32) to guide you through these steps.

What happens when you check all your favorite foods, and find each one is too high in fat? You have the opportunity to re-examine your taste preferences, your present body shape, your current weight, and your goals. If your preference for certain high fat foods and your goals are in conflict with each other, a choice has to be made. You have enough information and awareness by this time to make your food choices according to what you want for your future body.

Grams of Carbohydrate per Meal _____

COMPOSITION OF FOOD TABLE STANDARD PORTIONS 100 gms. or 3 1/2 oz.					PREFERRED FOOD LIST **CARBOHYDRATE**	MY USUAL PORTION IN gms. or oz.			
FOOD	CAL	PRO GMS	FAT GMS	CARB GMS	OZ./GMS	CAL	PRO GMS	FAT GMS	CARB GMS

Figure 27 - Preferred Food List for Carbohydrates

FOOD PORTION TABLE –

CARBOHYDRATE

AMOUNT OF FOOD IN OUNCES / GRAMS OF FAT	40	50	60	70	80	90	100	110
AVOCADO	20 oz / 100 g	25 oz / 125 g	30 oz / 150 g	35 oz / 175 g	40 oz / 200 g	45 oz / 225 g	50 oz / 250 g	55 oz / 275 g
BEANS, GREEN	32 oz / 0 g	40 oz / 1 g	48 oz / 2 g	56 oz / 3 g	64 oz / 4 g	72 oz / 5 g	80 oz / 6 g	88 oz / 7 g
BISCUITS W/EGGS, SHORTENING	3 oz / 15 g	3.5 oz / 17.5 g	4 oz / 20 g	5 oz / 25 g	6 oz / 30 g	6.5 oz / 32.5 g	7 oz / 35 g	7.5 oz / 37.5 g
BREAD, WHEAT	2 oz / 2 g	3 oz / 3 g	3.5 oz / 3.5 g	4 oz / 4 g	5 oz / 5 g	5.5 oz / 5.5 g	6 oz / 6 g	6.5 oz / 6.5 g
CORN CHIPS	2 oz / 13 g	2.5 oz / 16 g	3 oz / 19.5 g	3.5 oz / 23 g	4 oz / 26 g	4.5 oz / 29 g	5 oz / 32.5 g	5.5 oz / 36 g
COOKIES	2 oz / 12 g	2.5 oz / 15 g	3 oz / 18 g	3.5 oz / 21 g	4 oz / 24 g	4.5 oz / 27 g	5 oz / 30 g	5.5 oz / 33 g
CEREAL, FLAKES	2 oz / 2 g	2.2 oz / 2.2 g	2.6 oz / 2.6 g	3 oz / 3 g	3.5 oz / 3.5 g	4 oz / 4 g	4.2 oz / 4.2 g	4.6 oz / 4.6 g
MUFFINS, BAKERY	3 oz / 10 g	3.5 oz / 11 g	4 oz / 12 g	5 oz / 15 g	6 oz / 18 g	7 oz / 21 g	7.5 oz / 22 g	8 oz / 24 g
MUFFINS, HOME	3 oz / 4 g	4 oz / 6 g	5 oz / 7 g	5.5 oz / 7.5 g	6 oz / 9 g	7 oz / 10 g	8 oz / 12 g	9 oz / 13 g
OATS, DRY FORM	2 oz / 2 g	2.5 oz / 2.5 g	3 oz / 3 g	3.5 oz / 3.5 g	4 oz / 4 g	4.5 oz / 4.5 g	5 oz / 5 g	5.5 oz / 5.5 g
PANCAKES	4 oz / 8 g	5 oz / 10 g	6 oz / 12 g	7 oz / 14 g	8 oz / 16 g	9 oz / 18 g	10 oz / 20 g	11 oz / 22 g
PASTA, DRY FORM	2 oz / 1.2 g	2.5 oz / 1.5 g	2.7 oz / 1.7 g	3 oz / 2 g	3.2 oz / 2.2 g	3.5 oz / 2.5 g	3.7 oz / 2.7 g	4 oz / 3 g
PIZZA W/CHEESE	5 oz / 10 g	6 oz / 12 g	7 oz / 14 g	9 oz / 18 g	10 oz / 20 g	11 oz / 22 g	12 oz / 24 g	14 oz / 28 g
PIZZA W/O CHEESE	5 oz / 5 g	6 oz / 6 g	7 oz / 7 g	9 oz / 9 g	10 oz / 10 g	11 oz / 11 g	12 oz / 12 g	14 oz / 14 g
POPCORN, PLAIN	2 oz / 2 g	2.5 oz / 2.8 g	3 oz / 3.6 g	3.5 oz / 4.3 g	4 oz / 5 g	4.5 oz / 5.5 g	5 oz / 6 g	5.5 oz / 6.8 g
POPCORN, OIL & SALT	2.5 oz / 15 g	3 oz / 18 g	3.5 oz / 21 g	4 oz / 24 g	4.5 oz / 27 g	5 oz / 30 g	5.5 oz / 30 g	6 oz / 36 g
POTATO	7 oz / 0 g	8 oz / 0 g	10 oz / 0 g	11 oz / 0 g	13 oz / 0 g	14 oz / .1 g	16 oz / .2 g	17 oz / .3 g
RICE, DRY	6 oz / 0 g	7 oz / 0 g	8 oz / 0 g	10 oz / 0 g	11 oz / 0 g	12 oz / 0 g	14 oz / .1 g	15 oz / .2 g

Figure 28 - Food Portion Table for Carbohydrates

– GRAMS OF CARBOHYDRATE

120	130	140	150	160	170	180	190	200
60 oz / 300 g	65 oz / 325 g	70 oz / 350 g	75 oz / 375 g	80 oz / 400 g	85 oz / 425 g	90 oz / 450 g	95 oz / 475 g	100 oz / 500 g
96 oz / 8 g	104 oz / 9 g	112 oz / 10 g	120 oz / 11 g	128 oz / 12 g	136 oz / 13 g	144 oz / 14 g	152 oz / 15 g	160 oz / 16 g
8 oz / 40 g	9 oz / 45 g	10 oz / 50 g	10.5 oz / 52.5 g	11 oz / 55 g	12 oz / 60 g	12.5 oz / 62.5 g	13 oz / 65 g	14 oz / 70 g
7 oz / 7 g	8 oz / 8 g	8.5 oz / 8.5 g	9 oz / 9 g	10 oz / 10 g	10.5 oz / 10.5 g	11 oz / 11 g	11.5 oz / 11.5 g	12 oz / 12 g
6 oz / 39 g	6.5 oz / 42 g	7 oz / 45.5 g	7.5 oz / 48 g	8 oz / 52 g	8.5 oz / 55 g	9 oz / 58 g	9.5 oz / 61 g	10 oz / 65 g
6 oz / 36 g	6.5 oz / 39 g	7 oz / 42 g	87.5 oz / 45 g	8 oz / 48 g	8.5 oz / 51 g	9 oz / 54 g	9.5 oz / 57 g	10 oz / 60 g
5 oz / 5 g	5.5 oz / 5.5 g	6 oz / 6 g	6.2 oz / 6.2 g	6.6 oz / 6.6 g	7 oz / 7 g	7.5 oz / 7.5 g	8 oz / 8 g	8.2 oz / 8.2 g
9 oz / 27 g	10 oz / 30 g	10.5 oz / 32 g	11 oz / 33 g	12 oz / 36 g	13 oz / 39 g	13.5 oz / 41 g	14 oz / 42 g	15 oz / 45 g
10 oz / 15 g	10.5 oz / 15.5 g	11 oz / 16 g	12 oz / 18 g	13 oz / 19 g	14 oz / 21 g	14.5 oz / 21.5 g	15 oz / 22 g	16 oz / 24 g
6 oz / 6 g	6.5 oz / 6.5 g	7 oz / 7 g	7.5 oz / 7.5 g	8 oz / 8 g	8.5 oz / 8.5 g	9 oz / 9 g	9.5 oz / 9.5 g	10 oz / 10 g
12 oz / 24 g	13 oz / 26 g	14 oz / 28 g	15 oz / 30 g	16 oz / 32 g	17 oz / 34 g	18 oz / 36 g	19 oz / 38 g	20 oz / 40 g
4.2 oz / 3.2 g	4.5 oz / 3.5 g	4.7 oz / 3.7 g	5 oz / 4 g	5.2 oz / 4.2 g	5.5 oz / 4.5 g	5.7 oz / 4.7 g	6 oz / 5 g	6.2 oz / 5.2 g
15 oz / 30 g	16 oz / 32 g	17 oz / 34 g	19 oz / 38 g	20 oz / 40 g	21 oz / 42 g	22 oz / 44 g	24 oz / 48 g	25 oz / 50 g
15 oz / 15 g	16 oz / 16 g	17 oz / 17 g	19 oz / 19 g	20 oz / 20 g	21 oz / 21 g	22 oz / 22 g	24 oz / 24 g	25 oz / 25 g
6 oz / 7.2 g	6.5 oz / 7.8 g	7 oz / 8.4 g	7.5 oz / 9 g	8 oz / 9.6 g	8.5 oz / 10.2 g	9 oz / 10.8 g	9.5 oz / 11.4 g	10 oz / 12 g
6.5 oz / 39 g	7 oz / 42 g	7.5 oz / 45 g	8.5 oz / 48 g	8.5 oz / 51 g	9 oz / 54 g	9.5 oz / 57 g	10 oz / 60 g	10.5 oz / 63 g
19 oz / .4 g	20 oz / .5 g	21 oz / .6 g	22 oz / .7 g	24 oz / .8 g	25 oz / .9 g	27 oz / 1 g	28 oz / 1 g	30 oz / 1 g
16 oz / .3 g	18 oz / .4 g	19 oz / .5 g	20 oz / .6 g	22 oz / .7 g	23 oz / .8 g	24 oz / .9 g	26 oz / 1 g	27 oz / 1 g

Grams of Protein per Meal _____

COMPOSITION OF FOOD TABLE STANDARD PORTIONS 100 gms. or 3 1/2 oz.					PREFERRED FOOD LIST PROTEIN	MY USUAL PORTION IN gms. or oz.			
FOOD	CAL	PRO GMS	FAT GMS	CARB GMS	OZ./GMS	CAL	PRO GMS	FAT GMS	CARB GMS

Figure 29 - Preferred Food List for Protein

PROTEIN

FOOD PORTION TABLE — GRAMS OF PROTEIN

	AMOUNT OF FOOD IN OUNCES / GRAMS OF FAT	15 g	20 g	25 g	30 g	35 g	40 g	45 g	50 g
BEEF	CHOICE GRADE STEAK	2 oz / 6 g	3 oz / 8 g	4 oz / 10 g	5 oz / 12 g	6 oz / 14 g	7 oz / 16 g	8 oz / 18 g	9 oz / 20 g
	GROUND BEEF	3 oz / 18 g	4 oz / 24 g	5 oz / 29 g	6 oz / 36 g	7 oz / 42 g	8 oz / 48 g	9 oz / 54 g	10 oz / 60 g
DAIRY	MILK - 2%	13 oz / 8 g	17 oz / 12 g	21 oz / 13 g	25 oz / 15 g	30 oz / 10 g	33 oz / 20 g	38 oz / 23 g	42 oz / 25 g
	CHEDDAR CHEESE	2 oz / 19 g	3 oz / 26 g	4 oz / 36 g	4.5 oz / 40 g	5 oz / 45 g	6 oz / 54 g	6.5 oz / 59 g	7 oz / 64 g
	COTTAGE CHEESE - 2%	4 oz / 1 g	6 oz / 2 g	7 oz / 2 g	9 oz / 2 g	10 oz / 3 g	11 oz / 3 g	13 oz / 3 g	14 oz / 4 g
EGGS	WHOLE — RAW - EACH	2 / 14 g	3 / 21 g	4 / 28 g	4.5 / 32 g	5 / 35 g	6 / 42 g	6.5 / 46 g	7 / 49 g
	WHITES ONLY	4 / 0 g	5.5 / 0 g	6 / 0 g	8.5 / .0 g	10 / .0 g	11.5 / 0 g	12 / .0 g	13 / 0. g
FISH	HALIBUT — BROILED	2 oz / 4 g	3 oz / 6 g	4 oz / 8 g	4.5 oz / 9 g	5 oz / 10 g	6 oz / 12 g	6.5 oz / 13 g	7 oz / 14 g
	TUNA — IN OIL	2 oz / 13 g	3 oz / 19.5 g	3.5 oz / 22 g	4 oz / 26 g	4.5 oz / 29 g	5 oz / 32.5 g	6 oz / 39 g	6.5 oz / 42 g
	TUNA — IN WATER	2 oz / 1 g	2.5 oz / 1.2 g	3 oz / 1.5 g	3.5 oz / 1.7 g	4 oz / 2 g	4.5 oz / 2.2 g	5 oz / 2.5 g	6 oz / 2.7 g
PORK	BACON	1 oz / 15 g	1.5 oz / 20 g	2 oz / 26 g	2.3 oz / 31 g	2.6 oz / 35 g	3 oz / 40 g	3.3 oz / 45 g	3.6 oz / 49 g
	77% LEAN HAM	2 oz / 6 g	2.5 oz / 7.5 g	3 oz / 9 g	3.5 oz / 10.5 g	4 oz / 12 g	4.5 oz / 13.5 g	5 oz / 15 g	5.5 oz / 16.5 g
	PORK CHOPS	2 oz / 17 g	3 oz / 23 g	4 oz / 29 g	5 oz / 35 g	6 oz / 41 g	7 oz / 47 g	8 oz / 53 g	9 oz / 59 g
	SAUSAGE	3 oz / 33 g	4 oz / 44 g	5 oz / 55 g	6 oz / 66 g	7 oz / 77 g	8 oz / 88 g	9 oz / 99 g	10 oz / 110 g
POULTRY	CHICKEN WITH SKIN	2 oz / 6 g	2.5 oz / 7.5 g	3 oz / 9 g	3.5 oz / 10.5 g	4 oz / 12 g	4.5 oz / 13.5 g	5 oz / 15 g	5.5 oz / 16.5 g
	CHICKEN W/O SKIN	2 oz / 2 g	2.5 oz / 2.5 g	3 oz / 3 g	3.5 oz / 3.5 g	4 oz / 4 g	4.5 oz / 4.5 g	5 oz / 5 g	5.5 oz / 5.5 g
	TURKEY WITH SKIN	2 oz / 6 g	2.5 oz / 7.5 g	3 oz / 9 g	3.5 oz / 10.5 g	4 oz / 12 g	4.5 oz / 13.5 g	5 oz / 15 g	5.5 oz / 16.5 g
	TURKEY W/O SKIN	2 oz / 4 g	2.5 oz / 5 g	3 oz / 6 g	3.5 oz / 7 g	4 oz / 8 g	4.5 oz / 9 g	5 oz / 10 g	5.5 oz / 11 g
SEAFOOD	CRAB — STEAMED	3 oz / 3 g	4 oz / 4 g	5 oz / 5 g	6 oz / 6 g	7 oz / 7 g	8 oz / 8 g	9 oz / 9 g	10 oz / 10 g
	LOBSTER	3 oz / 2 g	4 oz / 2 g	5 oz / 3 g	6 oz / 3 g	7 oz / 4 g	8 oz / 4 g	9 oz / 5 g	10 oz / 5 g
	SHRIMP — BROILED/ STEAMED	3 oz / 1 g	4 oz / 1 g	5 oz / 1 g	6 oz / 1 g	7 oz / 1 g	8 oz / 2 g	9 oz / 2 g	10 oz / 2 g
MISCELLANEOUS	PEANUT BUTTER	2 oz / 28 g	3 oz / 42 g	4 oz / 56 g	4.5 oz / 63 g	5 oz / 70 g	6 oz / 84 g	7.5 oz / 91 g	7 oz / 98 g
	CASHEW NUTS	3 oz / 39 g	4 oz / 52 g	5 oz / 65 g	6 oz / 78 g	7 oz / 91 g	8 oz / 104 g	9 oz / 117 g	10 oz / 130 g

Figure 30 - Food Portion Table for Protein

How Much of "Your" Food Will You Need to Provide the Right Grams of Carbohydrates for Each Meal

STEP 1: Using the **FOOD PORTION TABLE** for carbohydrate foods (page 156), circle the grams of carbohydrates
you will eat per meal at the top of each column.

Example: 60 grams, potato

FOOD PORTION TABLE — GRAMS OF CARBOHYDRATES

AMOUNT OF FOOD IN OUNCES / GRAMS OF FAT	40	50	(60)	70	80	90	100	110
POTATO	7 oz / 0 g	8 oz / 0 g	9.5 oz / 0 g	11 oz / 0 g	13 oz / 0 g	14 oz / 0 g	16 oz / 0 g	17 oz / 0 g

STEP 2: Move down the column to a food you like
and note the amount of food needed ———————
and the amount of fat included in the food. ———

9.5 oz
0 g

STEP 3: Record the above information in your
PREFERRED FOOD LIST.

PREFERRED FOOD LIST — CARBOHYDRATE

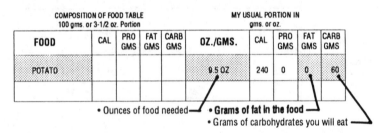

	COMPOSITION OF FOOD TABLE 100 gms. or 3-1/2 oz. Portion					MY USUAL PORTION IN gms. or oz.				
FOOD	CAL	PRO GMS	FAT GMS	CARB GMS	OZ./GMS.	CAL	PRO GMS	FAT GMS	CARB GMS
POTATO					9.5 OZ	240	0	0	60

• Ounces of food needed ⟋ • Grams of fat in the food ⟍
• Grams of carbohydrates you will eat ———

STEP 4: For the calorie amount - multiply carbohydrate grams by four, fat grams by nine, and, if protein is present, multiply by four.

EXAMPLE YOUR PORTION

Example: Carbohydrates:	60 grams x 4 calories/gms = 240 calories	_____ calories
Fat:	0 grams x 9 calories/gms = 0 calories	_____ calories
Protein:	_____ x 4 calories/gms = +0 calories	_____ calories

TOTAL: 240 Calories _____ Calories

NOTE: If one of your preferred foods is not listed in the Food Portion Table for carbohydrates, use the food tables at the end of the book to calculate your portion. (page 255) Record the table portions and your calculated portions in your Preferred Food List for future reference.

STEP 5: Weigh and prepare exactly the amount of the carbohydrate food, and notice the portion size. You will find it very useful to know what amount of space your portion of food occupies, for those times when a scale is not available.

Figure 31 - Example Directions for Carbohydrates

How Much of "Your" Food Will You Need to Provide the Right Grams of Protein for Each Meal

STEP 1:   Using the **FOOD PORTION TABLE** for protein foods (page 159), circle the grams of protein you will eat
per meal at the top of each column.

Example: 25 grams, chicken

FOOD PORTION TABLE – GRAMS OF PROTEIN

AMOUNT OF FOOD IN OUNCES / GRAMS OF FAT	15	20	⑤25	30	35	40	45	50
CHICKEN W/O SKIN	2 oz / 2 g	2.5 oz / 2.5 g	3 oz / 3 g	3.5 oz / 3.5 g	4 oz / 4 g	4.5 oz / 4.5 g	5 oz / 0 g	5.5 oz / 5.5 g

STEP 2:   Move down the column to a food you like
and note the amount of food needed ⟶ 3 oz
and the amount of fat included in the food. ⟶ 3 g

STEP 3:   Record the above information in your **PREFERRED FOOD LIST**.

PREFERRED FOOD LIST – PROTEIN

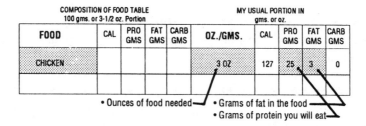

	COMPOSITION OF FOOD TABLE 100 gms. or 3-1/2 oz. Portion					MY USUAL PORTION IN gms. or oz.				
FOOD	CAL	PRO GMS	FAT GMS	CARB GMS	**OZ./GMS.**	CAL	PRO GMS	FAT GMS	CARB GMS
CHICKEN					3 OZ	127	25	3	0

• Ounces of food needed ⟶   • Grams of fat in the food ⟶
• Grams of protein you will eat ⟶

STEP 4:   For the calorie amount - multiply protein grams by four, fat grams by nine, and, if carbohydrate is present, multiply by four.

		EXAMPLE	YOUR PORTION

Example: Protein: 25 grams x 4 calories/gms = 100 calories _____ calories
                Fat: 3 grams x 9 calories/gms =   27 calories _____ calories
                Carbohydrate: _____ x 4 calories/gms =   +0 calories _____ calories

TOTAL: 127 Calories   _____ Calories

NOTE: If one of your preferred foods is not listed in the Food Portion Table for protein, use the food tables at the end of the book to calculate your portion. (page 255)
Record the table portions and your calculated portions in your Preferred Food List for future reference.

STEP 5:   Weigh and prepare exactly the amount of the protein food, and notice the portion size. You will find it very useful to know what amount of space your portion of food occupies, for those times when a scale is not available.

Figure 32 - Example Directions for Protein

Your personalized success program begins with Chapter One. All steps are based on your food preferences, goals and your Lean Body Mass. Consider the next eight steps as the foundation of your success plan with food. Fill in the charts provided as you progress.

1. Receive a body composition evaluation to determine your present pounds of LBM and fat. (Chapter 1)

2. Determine your vision and goals for your body. (Chapter 1)

3. Determine the number of calories you use per day based on your LBM and activities. (Chapters 2 & 4)

4. Choose the amount of calories you will eat per day. (Chapter 2)

5. Pick the percentages of protein, fat and carbohydrates calories you will use for your first six weex program. (Chapter 3)

6. Select the grams per meal from the Gram Conversion Table that match your percentage of each food component. (Chapter 3)

7. Pick the foods you like for the protein, fat and carbohydrate categories in the Composition of Foods Table. (Appendix 1)

8. Determine the amount of each food you need and fill in the following charts. (Figures 27 - 32, pp. 155 - 161)

You improve, and you are in control!

Wrapping Up

In each of the chapters so far, we have dealt with something that, in the past, was confusing or incomplete and stopped us from using food and training to achieve the weight, shape and performance we wanted. Each problem was followed by a new perspective for dealing with food and training. Notice that the Lean Body Mass is involved in every aspect of the solution.

Designing an effective individual food program requires that we examine our usual eating patterns. We must start with our vision and goals, and then include the basic information. In this case, the basic information is the LBM and the amount of proteins, fats, and carbohydrates in the food we like.

How to effectively include the new information daily requires a certain recipe. The recipe for each of us is unique and develops as we work with the planning process. The visual map on the next page is an excellent representation of what planning creates.

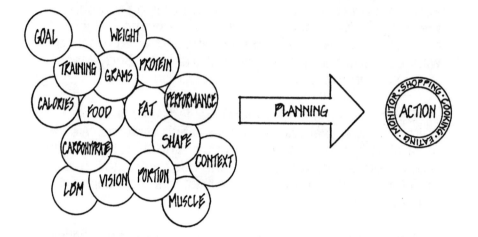

CHAPTER 6

Planning: From Knowledge to Action

"Modern technology has made everything available for
our improvement: equipment, exercise systems,
food plans, experts and monitoring devices.
And we continue to struggle with weight,
shape and energy level."

"Could the cause and solution to this struggle be linked
with our thoughts on what and how to eat?"

Overview

Chapter Six is a transition chapter, taking us from what we know about food, training and Lean Body Mass, to what action actually creates the results we want. Our standard approach is to skip from what we now know (Chapters 1-5) to "Let's Eat!" (Chapter 7).

There is one more ingredient that, when added, puts all the information into action within our schedules, so what we want will actually happen. The most critical and essential portion of the transition from what we know into action, and the source of power for making it happen, is "planning."

Planning is deliberately creating what you want. Planning is an ongoing learning experiment. Think about how much you will learn if you do a series of planned experiments, at two week intervals, for the next year. By planning your food and training for a two week period and monitoring with body compositions, you will have 26 opportunities during the next 52 weeks to learn and design your individualized program. The value of this chapter is in establishing a way to put all the information in the first five chapters together, before you proceed to Chapter Seven, Shopping, Cooking, and Eating.

New Food Concepts

Common sense and creativity will be the approach to food and eating in Chapters Six and Seven. One of the basic concepts is to experiment. Outstanding results come from experimenting with all aspects of your food program.

My plan is to have these next few paragraphs give you total permission to be creative, and experiment with your food. Each experiment will have a definite result. The freedom to experiment comes with the responsibility to monitor the result. We have been experimenting for years with food, anyway, under the disguise of diets, new recipes and many other plans for eating. We have created changes in our body weight and shape by not being aware of our food, and now, perhaps, it is time to control the process.

As you become more innovative with food within your range of percentages for protein, fats and carbohydrates, you will find an infinite variety of tastes, food combinations, and varying amounts of food that will fit into your improvement program. I have found, from thousands of diet surveys, that people tend to eat the same foods, with very little variety week after week. This new process will not only establish variety and creativity, it will have a dramatic effect on your rate of improvement.

Thinking Protein and Carbohydrates

Miracles happen when people begin to think of foods, meal plans, shopping, cooking and eating, in terms of protein and carbohydrates rather than food and eating. Thinking of food in terms of carbohydrates and protein is similar to thinking of the body in terms of muscle and Lean Body Mass. The first advantage of this thought process is that a decision about what to eat is automatic.

Usually, when planning a meal or ordering in a restaurant, we think in terms of the meat or fish first. Carbohydrates, the main portion of your meal, are almost an afterthought; and the fat portion of the meal, which we want to minimize, is not considered to be a factor, and is usually included in excess.

The major strategy suggested, one that works for your body and your meals, is to start with the question, "Which carbohydrates do I want?" What comes to mind is your carbohydrate food, (for example, rice) and the approximate amount your body needs per meal (for example, 85 grams or 2 cups). The next question is, "Which proteins do I want?" The answer is selected from your preferred protein choices, in the appropriate amount to support your Lean Body Mass and goals.

Please notice this is an entirely different approach to eating, and is based on foods you like that match your Lean Body Mass and goals, rather than on random foods that satisfy hunger.

Separating and Combining Foods

Once you identify your favorite carbohydrate and protein foods, you can begin one of the more important steps for your improvement: That is, specifically separating carbohydrates from proteins. By "separating", I am referring to having carbohydrates for one meal and protein for the next. The main concern when separating carbohydrates and proteins is inconvenience, because we will have to eat differently than we always have. Perhaps, eating the way we always have has limited our improvement in the past. At this point, most of us should welcome an opportunity to be creative with our food program in a way that lets us alter our weight and shape.

To begin, carbohydrates and proteins are digested differently. Protein digestion occurs within the stomach in an acid environment. Carbohydrate digestion begins in the mouth, continues in the stomach in a neutral to alkaline environment, and is finished in the small intestine. When people separate these foods at least one meal each day, a more rapid change in body composition is observed.

Eating carbohydrates at one meal and protein at another does not mean carbohydrates for breakfast, and protein for lunch. This could result in too few calories, with the protein and carbohydrate foods spaced too far apart. This particular eating pattern means, as an example: carbohydrates for breakfast, protein mid-morning; carbohydrates for lunch, and protein mid-afternoon. Review the concept of experimenting before you determine that this particular program is not possible. (Also, at this time, I would encourage you, as a reader, to set aside all thoughts and reservations about how you'll prepare the food, what food it will be, how it could be packaged, and how convenient it will be. This will be covered in Chapter 7.)

The interval between eating carbohydrates and eating proteins should be two to three hours. In many situations, it will not be possible to eat carbohydrates and proteins at two separate times. This might occur when eating away from home, or when you have a schedule that does not allow the separation. If we usually eat three meals per day and 21 meals a week, I am certain there will be many opportunities to plan your food program to include a number of meals with carbohydrates and proteins two to four hours apart.

There are foods that can be eaten together and are processed by the body in the stomach and small intestine efficiently. There are also foods that, when eaten in combination, actually impair the digestion of each other.

The following is a review of food-combining basics:

1. Eat fruit or fruit juice first; 15 minutes before, or two hours after, your meal. Fruit is digested differently and at a much faster rate. It can interfere with the digestion of other food.

2. Desserts, like fruit, should be eaten before your meal for similar reasons. Remember when you were younger and wanted to always eat dessert first?

3. A suggestion: As mentioned earlier, the beginning process of digestion for carbohydrates (your most important food) starts in the mouth. Chew your food! Your body will appreciate the effort and reward you by digesting more and storing less of it as fat.

Symptoms of poor food combining are: gastric upset, belching, acid indigestion, intestinal gas, cramping, and varying degrees of diarrhea and constipation. It has always been fascinating to me that the standard cure for gastric upset, due to the way in which we combine and eat our foods, is to eat antacids. Consuming antacids to neutralize our poor food combining, while the stomach is attempting to correct the problem, doesn't make a great deal of sense, unless you are the one selling the antacids.

Many people say they would rather eat the way they always have, combine the foods that don't work, and follow the meal with Tums, Di-Gel or Rolaids, than do something different. In this case, they are asking the entire body to suffer the consequences of food which may be toxic to our system simply because of the taste. It is quite possible that what we always do with food may cause many of the problems or symptoms we would like to correct.

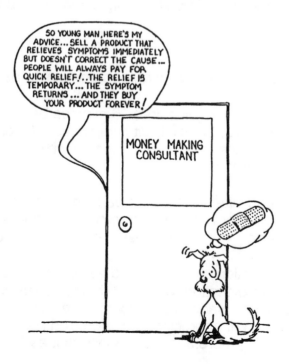

Food combining is the subject of many books. For the sake of simplicity, we will say:

1. Combine salads and proteins.

2. Combine salads and carbohydrates.

3. Eat fruits separately, because of their unique processing by the body.

Symptoms and Food

How we eat could have everything to do with certain headache problems, cravings, allergies, low blood sugar, water retention, hunger and low metabolism. How we eat takes into account not just the type of protein or carbohydrate, but also the balance of proteins and carbohydrates, undereating and overeating, and the combination and separation of certain foods.

Headaches. Headaches that are not on one side of the head or the other, and which occur almost daily in a person of any age (especially children), are not due to a deficiency in aspirin or other pain medication. Some people will spend months and even years trying different types of pain medication, believing that they have not yet found the right chemical for their particular pain pattern. Headaches are not a natural phenomenon. The following are three examples of the more common food patterns that result in headaches.

1. Not eating regularly, and not eating enough, results in headaches and low blood sugar.

2. Frequent consumption of a standard food, such as dairy products, may cause an allergy headache.

3. Certain foods eaten in combination, such as steak and melon, for example, can cause headaches and other problems, which will not occur when these foods are eaten separately.

It makes sense, is less expensive, and is far more rewarding to experiment with food as the cause of a problem for a week or two, rather than spend months and years taking pain medication. If our first thought when a headache occurs was, "Could this be food related?", rather than, "Where's the aspirin?", there would be less pain patterns. Headaches that persist could be more accurately and quickly treated by health care professionals.

Cravings and Addictions. Most of us think cravings for certain foods or substances, and addictions are something other people have. One client answered my question about his craving and addiction for sugar with the classic comment, "I never crave sugar; I have it all the time!" Chocolate, tobacco, alcohol, sugar, caffeine, other foods, and even some non-food related cravings, sometimes have interesting common sense solutions. Doesn't it raise a question in your mind about food, and its influence on us, when you learn one of the main solutions for cravings, headaches, low blood sugar, and allergies is related to balancing carbohydrates and proteins to your individual body?

Low Blood Sugar. Being emotional, grouchy, irritable, hungry, or having headaches and stomach cramps are a few symptoms of low blood sugar. Low blood sugar, or hypoglycemia, is not a disease, but a symptom. The cause could be any one of a combination of the following: not eating, or eating high sugar substances, caffeine or using tobacco. In all instances, the blood sugar level will rise for a short period of time, and then drop below normal.

Earlier in the book, we discussed carbohydrates as the main energy source for our muscles and brain. Carbohydrates are stored as muscle glycogen and glucose or blood sugar . Glucose circulates at a certain level in the blood, and is available to muscle tissue and brain cells at all times. Blood sugar levels which are higher or lower than normal can cause multiple symptoms, which can mimic other illness patterns.

We all experience changes in blood sugar levels at different times of the day. The objective is to maintain a normal and stable level for optimum mental and physical performance and emotional stability. We have enough stress to occupy us at any given moment, so why not have our food be a support system, rather than a part of the stress pattern we deal with daily? The solution to blood sugar level problems is food, and the cause of this problem is food. Fortunately, the way in which we describe eating will not only work for your lean mass, weight and shape; it will also resolve blood sugar level problems.

Allergies. Allergies are always described to us in terms of symptoms, such as a stuffy nose, watery eyes or rash. Even water retention can be a symptom of the body's allergic reaction to a certain kind of food. These symptoms, are the result of the body's reaction to foreign protein called allergens. Allergens come from a food which cannot be broken down by the body's digestive enzymes, or a substance that cannot be resisted by the body's immune system. When the immune system can no longer fight or resist the allergen, the symptom becomes obvious. Long before the stuffy nose becomes apparent, the body's systems have been engaged in a 24-hour-a-day battle for months, and sometimes years.

If the body is allergic to a common food eaten daily (wheat, meat, dairy, or chocolate), the body's immune and enzyme systems stay busily engaged in fighting this enemy. Under these conditions, any outside allergen, such as dust or pollen, can appear to be the culprit. In reality, a food substance to which we are allergic can weaken the immune system. Until that is taken care of, we are susceptible to other influences, which under normal conditions would not cause a reaction.

Learning to separate and combine foods will allow people to begin to identify possible allergic foods.

Low Metabolism. When the body cannot burn enough calories to keep weight under control, and the person is inactive and has a low energy level, the diagnosis is often low metabolism. The treatment is a chemical which speeds up the body's metabolism. If low metabolism was thought of as a symptom, the approach and solution would change.

Observing low metabolism as a symptom requires a different line of questioning to explain the cause. Without exception, each person with a low metabolism will have a substantial decrease in Lean Body Mass--the part of the body responsible for metabolism. It would be beneficial for us to determine why the Lean Body Mass has decreased, and what type of program would re-establish it and increase metabolism.

Hunger. The bottom line for the majority of us is this: When the blood sugar level drops, we get hungry! We are not plants, and do not get energy from water, air, or sunshine. Our brains and bodies demand carbohydrates, protein, and a small amount of fat. When these substances are not provided, especially carbohydrates and protein, our body breaks down muscle tissue to feed itself and obtain energy for growth and repair. Our bodies cannot make carbohydrates or protein from fat.

This is a reminder that our bodies have specific needs, regardless of age or size or energy level; and those needs, are specific to each individual. The amount of food we need in each category is unique to each person; yet, we all need carbohydrates in a range from 50% to 65%, proteins in a range from 15% to 25%, and fats in a range from 10% to 25%.

The question, "How do we deal with hunger?" becomes, "How do we deal with hunger and not gain weight?" The answer to this question, and the solution to the symptoms of headaches, allergies, cravings, low blood sugar, controlling weight and shape, losing fat, and adding Lean Body Mass while increasing your energy level, is the same. The solution and the answer is simply food. What we eat, how much we eat, and how we separate our food can be an answer to symptoms that have plagued us for years. However, when a food plan is offered as a solution to the problems we have had for years, there is still reluctance to accept it, because anything new requires change. There are multiple reasons, blocks, and barriers to actually starting and continuing a better food program, even when it is obvious that the new program will work.

Solving the Mystery

What is more complicated than food? There is a great deal of controversy and opinion involved in every aspect of this topic. When food programs are based on theories and opinions, there will always be confusion. When food programs are based on our Lean Body Mass, the confusion can stop! There will be less argument about which diet is right, and which expert has the best technique. Then there will be a race to see who can inspire people to improve in the most efficient manner, within each individual's lifestyle and goals.

When health care reaches this level, it will not be a matter of which program works best. There will only be one program, and that will be to balance the carbohydrates, proteins and fats. Once health care professionals and fitness experts become clear about the balance of foods and food components, their focus will be on support for the client. In other words, all experts will join forces for one concept that will fit the goals of people, and create the desired results. This concept will take away the right and wrong of a program, and focus on people improving, rather than on something insignificant, such as, "My program is better than your program."

Impatience. Even after reducing much of the mystery about food, explaining the relationship between food and Lean Body Mass, using charts and graphs, and even allowing people to select their own food, there is still resistance because of old habits, unwillingness to change, and inconvenience. One of the common complaints is that losing fat is too slow. The fat loss rate for women is usually slower than for men, because women have a lower amount of Lean Body Mass.

EXAMPLE

Woman - 130 lbs	**Man** - 180 lbs
LBM - 90 lbs	LBM - 140 lbs
Fat - 40 lbs	FAT - 40 lbs
35% Muscle = 31 lbs	**45% Muscle = 63 lbs**

Notice that the male has approximately two times the muscle mass of the female. This is not meant to discourage the female population about weight change. It is meant to explain, and to let you know why change happens slower for the female, why they require more patience, and why an increase in exercise, and even more exactness with food, could be necessary. The other message is to stop comparing our rate of change with another person's rate of change. How fast we change depends on our Lean Body Mass, and about three or four hundred other factors. Comparing does not create answers. The awareness of LBM has helped influence how many people feel about their amount of muscle tissue, and how valuable this part of their body really is.

Barriers to Planning

A subtle barrier to planning occurs when you feel using LBM and grams is complicated. This conversion requires a short adjustment period. By keeping your focus on the results you want for your future body, you will stay motivated through these first few weeks.

A common interruption of the planning process is family members. They are concerned that their favorite foods and treats will be eliminated. The same family recipes that everyone enjoys can also be prepared to satisfy both your food requirements, and goals for your body. Plan to leave out the fat in your traditional recipes. It is a challenge that will benefit everyone for life.

Another barrier to actually starting a new approach for food is the belief that, "If I eat differently, my friends wouldn't understand!" My response to these people is consistent. I explain that our friends understand great bodies; we all do. Try being the first on your block to create a new body, and no one will notice that you eat differently. They will, however, notice you!

Occasionally, the new information, body composition evaluations, and the number of years the person has struggled with weight and shape, is still not enough incentive to change. It takes tremendous strength and commitment for a person who has not ever worked with a new training or food program to improve for the first time. In this situation, success can be achieved by working with a coach or advisor.

The Incentive to Begin a New Food Program

What seems to work consistently in helping people create an unshakeable foundation for their new personal program is, an understanding of their personal blocks and barriers in the area of food and training. We often discover that what stops us in this area is the same process that stops us in other situations. Once we recognize the barriers, we can begin to organize a support system of friends, family and coaches to guarantee our success.

One person with a desire to change weight and shape can create an opportunity for many people to improve. One motivated person can cause enough interest in the fitness and healthcare community to establish body composition evaluations, bring in speakers, and develop support groups.

Here is an interesting concept that helps people establish a financial value for their Lean Body Mass. The grocery store price for protein varies from six dollars to ten dollars per pound. Notice the quality of the meat, poultry or seafood being displayed, according to its percent of muscle and fat. Now determine the price of *your* muscle per pound. One pound could be worth hundreds of thousands of dollars depending on your lifetime value. How would you care for a piece of equipment that was this valuable? My guess is that you would not only keep it in the best possible condition, you would want to show it off to your friends.

Consistently using body composition evaluations always works to maintain motivation and incentive for people to be certain the muscle is being maintained. Motivation to continue comes from the results people see when they keep track of food and training, and keep an accurate journal of their progress and procedures.

The Motivation to Continue

The best part about training and eating according to your Lean Body Mass is that you are designing your own program, your own pace, and your own rate of change. There are some rules and suggestions that will, if applied, create fun and personal satisfaction as you move towards your goals. The rules include: permission to be creative; a summary of the correct amount of food; how many calories to eat; what type of food to eat; making the program fun and interesting; food combination; and what to do about the "wrong" foods.

Although there is a great deal of technology throughout this book regarding fat loss, you have absolute permission and total freedom to do or not do any of the procedures. With this system you can always win-- slowly or rapidly--over a long or short period of time. Once you have experienced progress, and your improvement lapses for a time, you can always use your individualized plan to recreate the body composition scores you like.

Body composition evaluations encourage you to become absolutely honest about your activity and food. Without the evaluation as a motivator, it is impossible to know how well your program is working. So, by firmly establishing your goals and scheduling body compositions ahead of time, you have given yourself permission to win!

Food To Fit Your Body

Food has been, and will continue to be, reviewed from every aspect because of its importance to our weight and shape control. It might be interesting to pay as much attention to how food fits our body as we do to how clothes fit our body. The charts, tables and summary in Chapter Five will help remind you of your preferred foods.

What Type of Food can I Eat?

1. Begin by being aware of the foods you normally eat. Notice the amount of protein, carbohydrate and fat in these foods.

2. For a maximum change, begin recording the amounts of protein, carbohydrate and fat in your meals.

3. Accurate recording will give you a clear idea of where to make changes in your food program after your next body composition evaluation.

How Often Should I Eat?

1. Food molecules (nutrients) are absorbed by the cells of the body for two to six hours after you have eaten the food. Then, depending upon the type of food consumed, the body is ready for another supply of fuel two to six hours after a meal.

2. The body will process small amounts of food in frequent meals throughout the day better than a large amount all at once toward the end of the day.

3. The body prefers a constant supply of nutrients from high quality foods rather than an inconsistent supply due to random feedings.

4. Eat a minimum of three meals per day. Eating three meals a day does not necessarily allow for separating carbohydrates and proteins. I suggest that initially a person use one meal per day in which he or she separates carbohydrates and proteins. For most people, it is a challenge to schedule three well balanced meals a day. Separating carbohydrates and protein for one meal may be viewed as an inconvenience, and it is also the first step you can take in creating your future body.

Making it Fun and Interesting

1. Change your eating program or change the proportions of protein, carbohydrate and fat every six weeks. The body adapts to food plans, which causes progress to slow. Program modification reduces this tendency and eliminates boredom.

2. Add at least one new meal plan to your program every week for variety. Write these in your journal for future reference.

3. Schedule "fun" meals, if you like. Three meals per day equals twenty-one meals per week. That means, eat whatever you want, and as much as you like, after you have satisfied your protein and carbohydrate requirements. Eventually, you will get tired of two free-for-all meals per week, and plan for only one. I find it quite interesting that these particular eating sessions lose their appeal after a few months.

The reason for fun meals is not very complicated. It allows for dinner out, a few extra desserts, or just eating a large amount. These actions help to convince your mind that you are not being punished. This system removes the concept of denial. Your body will not store all the calories from this one meal. It is essential to return immediately to your eating program, following the fun meal.

Keep these meals as far apart as possible. Example: Sunday brunch and Wednesday dinner. It will be interesting, and you will look forward to these mini celebrations. Your fun meal is the second or third meal of the day. It is absolutely critical that you do not skip meals on this day.

How Soon Will I See A Change?

You body composition evaluation may reveal a change in your body long before you can see it. Changes happen sooner under the following conditions:

1. You agree to eat according to the LBM chart and intake sheets. If you undereat, your body will not do what you expect.

2. You keep an accurate record of food intake and activity level. What we actually eat and what we *think* we eat are often not the same.

3. Change occurs when you consume 200 to 800 calories per day less than you burn, depending primarily upon your activity level and size. One rule to follow is to never go below your base calories.

4. One pound of fat contains approximately 3600 calories. Fat is burned in the muscle tissue when the muscle is stimulated by movement. Losing one pound of fat per week is rapid for most of us.

5. If you use more calories than you eat, and your food is balnced to your LBM, your body will use some stored body fat. One pound of fat equals 3600 calories. If you use 500 extra calories per day, you can lose one pound of fat every ten to fourteen days. (Not all the calories we use each day are fat calories.)

6. Often, a person will lose much more than one pound of *scale weight* per week. In this case, a allergy food was probably eliminated. These foods tend to cause water retention and, consequently, a majority of the weight loss is water. When this happens, I encourage the person to identify the food or beverage which caused the allergy.

The "Wrong" Food: A New Value System

Some factors that influence our decisions about foods are: where we are; what we have time for; what is available; the cost of the food; what our mouth wants; what our body wants; and what is our goal. One more question needs to be addressed, which is, "What about wrong foods?"

Including the Wrong Food

Defining foods as good or bad, right or wrong, does not work as well as asking the question, "Will this food create the result I want?" A great deal of our available food has been processed, or changed in some way, to improve the taste. When nutrition or health-oriented people talk about bad foods, they are usually met with universal resistance. We are thinking of health; most people are thinking of taste. It is the obligation of the food industry to make food taste good. Therefore, the responsibility for dealing with the processed and fat foods (which taste "good") belongs to you. Even the good foods included on your "preferred foods" list can cause some problems, if eaten in excess of your portions.

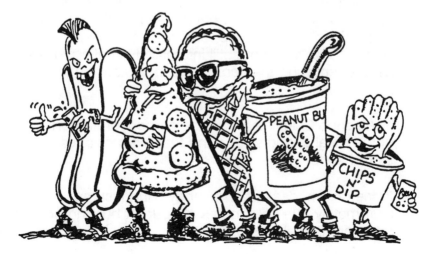

What causes certain foods to be a "wrong" food?

- The processing concentrates the calories, and makes the food hard to digest; this confuses the body's systems. It is far better to eat foods that contain their own necessary nutrients for processing, than to eat processed foods which have excess calories.

- Undesirable foods include fat in excessive amounts. Excess calories are those over the amount the body can process per meal. The excess calories we eat in the form of fat, protein or carbohydrate are converted into excess body fat.

Another major problem is the over-consumption of refined carbohydrates. Throughout this book, I have emphasized complex carbohydrates as a main energy supply for brain and muscles. Refined carbohydrates have been chemically changed, or processed in ways to make them taste sweeter and cook faster.

Foods that Don't Support our Goals

The first and most important step is to learn how many grams of protein, carbohydrate and fat the food contains. Weigh it; look it up; and write it down prior to eating the food. If you are still interested in eating these foods after knowing their composition, review the following:

1. Alcohol: Calculate it into the carbohydrate portion of the meal and keep in mind that extra calories get stored as fat.

2. Ice cream, dessert and candy: Run first, approximately 10 - 15 minutes at your fat burning heart rate per 100 calories of food.

3. Pizza: Consider an experiment. Order half of your pizza without cheese. All of the fat is in the cheese. One piece with cheese can cancel out a 30 to 40 minute workout.

4. Nuts, seeds, cheese and avocados: Look up the fat content; it is unbelievable. Weigh the amount you are going to eat, and do the same thing when eating ice cream and candy.

5. Pasta: a carbohydrate, not a wrong food. It is the meat and cheese sauces that contain the fat--not the pasta.

6. Finally, if you are really going to eat them, eat all these foods at one time, in one meal, and your body will store less of it. Then get back to the proportions, and foods that will help you reach your goal.

When you have taken the responsibility to calculate and learn the components of an undesirable food, the mystery and power of that food seem to go away. Once you know what that food is made of, you have a choice: to eat the food or not to eat the food! Knowing eliminates surprises. A major problem occurs when you choose not to find out what is in the food. This decision relates directly to the two concepts upon which this book is based: personal choice and your optimum performance.

The Key to Winning

Planning Overview. Planning our food meals and menus involves everything we need to satisfy our Lean Body Mass, energy and fat loss requirements. The meal plan is really a mini version of how we plan our food for the day, month or even year. Ultimately, the composition of food eventually equals the composition of our body. The design and planning of an eating program must be based on what we want to look like years from now, rather than what will satisfy our mouths for a few seconds. Properly planned food can satisfy our goals for our body, as well as, our request for great tasting food.

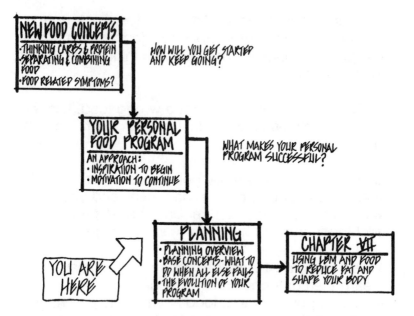

Why Have a Five to Ten Year Goal. In setting a five to ten year goal, we disregard age, because muscles do not know how old they are. Muscles only perform. With proper food and activity, muscles perform consistently. Five to ten year goals are written according to what we want to accomplish with more energy and less fat, instead of simply being ten years older, with less energy than we now have. This would be an ideal time to list what you want for weight, Lean Body Mass and fat, body measurements, and performance in the future.

Establishing a One-year Goal. I have noticed we fit food and training into our lives much more easily when we plan. The result of planning is that a project is accomplished. Can you imagine a building or ship being constructed without a plan and a schedule? The end result of the project would be vague or nonexistent. The majority of us qualify as members of a group that have built their bodies without a long-term plan.

The new perspective in planning is that we become the "planner." We design and plan the food and training process with our own goals, schedules and preferences in mind. For some people, being in charge means there is no one else to blame, the excuses are taken away, and what is left is their own responsibility. For most of us, designing our own program is a freedom from the old habits and the beliefs that we could never control weight and shape.

Establishing a one-year goal begins the process of creating your future body. The random approach, without a plan for food and activity, has resulted in your present body weight, shape and performance. If you choose to improve, a goal is required. The muscles are unaware of your age, and will respond to the activity and food you provide. So why not choose goals worthy of your LBM; goals that will help you get where you really want to be? What you accomplish, and where you will be in five to ten years, starts with your one-year goal. Having the body you want is worth the planning process.

When planning for the year, record all events you know will occur. Then write in the possibilities for training and other activities for the different seasons. In line with planning the year, there will also be certain events or trips you want to create. This would be the time to write them into your one-year plan. You can also have other shorter term goals regarding meetings or classes. These would be included in your one-year goal.

Keeping the ten year and lifetime goal in mind, let's look specifically at the next twelve months from the standpoint of body composition.

Step 1: Determine from the present what you want in one year.

	ONE YEAR	ONE MONTH	ONE WEEK
Weight:			
LBM:			
Fat:			

Step 2: Creating a monthly plan. Keeping the one-year goal in mind, the month goal will be simply 1/12th of the yearly plan. Just as in establishing the yearly goal, write in all activities, meetings, celebrations, and body composition evaluations that you have already scheduled, and that you want to include during the month. Our main emphasis will be on the weekly and daily schedules which, of course, are a representation of your month program.

Step 3: Establishing your one-week goal. The details and the chart for your one-week planning process is explained and illustrated in Chapter Seven.

1. Plan the number of meals per week that will be composed of both proteins and carbohydrates, the number of meals that will be carbohydrates alone, and the number of meals per week that will be protein alone. These meals will be planned ahead of time.

2. Plan the training sessions ahead of time, and include them in the weekly schedule.

3. Plan the food program (eating schedule) ahead of time, and include in the week's schedule.

Before the week has started, you will have the training schedule in place, meals scheduled, calories per day and the amounts of your favorite foods listed. What is left for you to do is shop for, prepare and eat the food. Chapter Seven takes care of shopping and cooking. Your last bit of homework will be to relax, grin and improve as you eat.

Other Considerations

Let's consider that each week starts with Saturday. This not only breaks the monotony of starting on Mondays, it allows us an entirely different focus on our time schedule. Because of the traditional "Monday start," we have convinced ourselves that we deserve to rest on weekends. This means we take a break and eat whatever we want, as a reward.

By starting our week with Saturday, we find two extra days to design meals, prepare food and design training into the rest of the week. Our intention is to create the schedule for our week and month, rather than start Monday, and hope that somehow during the week we have time to squeeze in some training, and eat when we can.

The goal is to plan your day as a model of your week, and have your week represent your month. So, if we multiply your monthly schedule by twelve, you would have a program that would work for an entire year. There is great flexibility in your food program by substituting carbohydrates and proteins, and equal flexibility in your training program by substituting different activities. Continue to monitor your progress every two to four weeks with a body composition evaluation.

Menus and Meals

All families and individuals have personal food and taste preferences. It is always possible to design menus and meals that fit the body's requirements. The challenge is to design meals that fit people's taste requirements.

After reading through Chapters One to Five, and learning in theory all about food and planning, we are still faced with the practical question of what to do each day for each meal.

Considering that we eat approximately 1,000 meals per year, the planning, cooking and eating can occupy much of our time and decision-making processes. It's no wonder we get very tired of preparing meals and deciding what to eat. Who has the energy to rethink our meals each time? We become easy prey to outside influences, such as fast food, and inside influences, such as low blood sugar.

It is relatively easy to become overwhelmed with planning meals. There are so many variables regarding eating, that having a plan lets us be easily in control during any of the following situations.

Variables that Influence our Food Choices

What Type of Food: commercial, packaged, heat-and-eat, homemade and natural.

Where to Eat: home, away from home, school, work, traveling, entertainment and vacation.

Time of Day: morning, mid-day, evening, weekdays and weekends.

How Much Food: number of meals per day, the right amount per meal.

Who Knows: which expert, which diet, which method of training, which book.

Considering all of the above variables, it becomes quite a challenge to juggle the food requirement for our own busy lives, not to mention taking care of a family. Within all this potential confusion, if we could have one basic rule, or answer, to fall back on when our schedules and decisions get crazy, one language that answers all of these variables and considerations, we might find some peace in the world of the food decisions we make every day.

The answer or language is not to be found in special diets, from experts, or as a result of different opinions. The way to organize and design food that fits all the variables is to use the balance of proteins, carbohydrates and fats to fit your LBM and activity!

With a balance of food components as the base, the key is to think protein and carbohydrates, rather than, "I'm hungry; what's the most convenient food?" While "protein and carbohydrates" does not seem like much of an answer to the question, "What should I eat?", it points you in a direction where you can find answers that fit your individual preference and schedule.

This is how thinking "protein and carbohydrates" could be an answer to the variables listed above.

Type of Food: All foods can now be thought of, and placed in a category of either protein or carbohydrates. At this point the food has to satisfy your body's requirements, in addition to your hunger.

Where to Eat: Whether we are at home or away, thinking in terms of proteins and carbohydrates always works. If our goal is to change body composition, eating away from home can be the same as eating at home.

Time of Day: Any food can be used for any meal, from a protein and carbohydrate standpoint, as long as it fits within the stated requirements and goals.

How Much Food: The amounts of protein and carbohydrate in the foods you like have already been decided and calculated. There is no longer an excuse for not knowing how much to eat.

Who Knows: All books, diets and experts have something of value to offer. Now you can take their information, and select the portion that fits your goal and your food program, while keeping in mind your body's personal requirements.

From my experience, every problem, consideration, obstacle and question people have had in this area was solved by basing the grams per day on the Lean Body Mass, and balancing their percentage of proteins, fats and carbohydrates.

The Evolution of Your Personal Food Plan

Today there is great concern, regarding chemicals, steroids and other additives in the food we eat. There is equal concern regarding the effects of processed versus whole foods. It would be important to have a basic plan, philosophy or approach to use when considering an overall food program. These steps allow people to use a new approach with their belief system; or allow them to adapt their belief systems to any new approach.

1. Macronutrients. Macronutrients, the foundation of a food program, are the correct amounts of protein, fat and carbohydrate for each person, according to the LBM, training program and goals. I am suggesting this food plan as a replacement for the basic four food groups, which have long been used as the standard and are incomplete when used alone.

It is a time for replacement. A concept that works is needed, something that is universal and gives freedom and latitude to food plans. Adaptability, lack of fat, consideration of allergic foods, and food combining--which are often lacking in the basic four--is automatically in place when balancing the basic macronutrients: proteins, fats and carbohydrates.

2. Processed Versus Whole Food. Once you understand the balance and combination of macro components, it will be important to begin learning and experimenting with processed versus whole foods. As the number of processed foods and additives increases, and foods are sprayed with more chemicals, the issue of internal environmental control may become as popular, and generate as much concern as the pollution of our external environment. Perhaps internal and external are not separate, and must be solved simultaneously.

3. Micronutrients. Micronutrients are vitamins, minerals, fiber and water. It has been demonstrated, without question, that processing and refining food removes vitamins, minerals and fiber, which are necessary for many of the body processes. Even our non-processed foods are often lacking in micronutrients; because of decreased nutrients in the soil, because foods are no longer brought directly from the field to our table, and as a result of preserving methods used for shipping. The important message is to be responsible for knowing that the deficiency exists, and consider adding these micronutrients to your already balanced macronutrient food plan. Macronutrients are necessary for the absorption of the vitamin and mineral component of the micronutrients.

Most of our choices regarding which food plan we will use are based on our minds, research data, a diet plan, or a motive such as losing weight. There is a tendency to disregard, or not be aware of, how our body is tolerating our intellectual choice of food. At the present time, the most valuable communication link we have with our body is the body composition evaluation. Any change in food is an experiment, and may or may not work for your body. When experimenting with how your body receives the macronutrients, I would advise consistent body composition evaluations to monitor your vital lean mass to fat ratio. As we have said many times, the body knows more about your food program than your mind, and will respond accordingly.

Wrapping Up

There are very few aspects of our life that are as personal and consistent as the food ritual. Belief systems and opinions concerning food are always quite strong and reinforced with every meal. No one should change a familiar food program, unless there is a concern about weight, shape, energy level, or performance. Then a change in how we eat is necessary.

Any change in how we eat will not last long unless it includes our own taste preferences. A change in diet must be convincing and effective, or there is discouragement, and we go back to our old eating habits. After all, if nothing works we might as well eat the food we like.

If we are going to make a change in our eating pro-gram, we want it to create results we like. Once we know what we want, planning begins to answer the question, "How are we going to make it happen?"

The planning process means creating your future self, on purpose. Our future self is being created, and will hap-pen anyway on the basis of what we are doing or not doing; just like tomorrow, next week and next year will happen anyway, with or without us. We can be passive spectators and hope tomorrow will be a "good" day, or at least not a "bad" one, or we can be active participants, schedule in a great day, and see how close we come to our expectations. In the participant mode, we can make any necessary corrections and plan the next day. What better method to experiment with than food and training?

Planning, in the context of food and our bodies, is a future-oriented activity. It is living life "on purpose," creat-ing "ahead of time," and then comparing what happened to what we said would happen. A minimum amount of time is spent on historical data, with the major focus on the planning process that will match what we want for next week, next year--and our new body.

Planning does not remove choices and creativity, especially in the arena of LBM. It actually opens new creative possibilities for your schedule, food, body and training. The planning process includes all data, informa-tion, experience and recordkeeping, and then designs the map for shopping, cooking and eating.

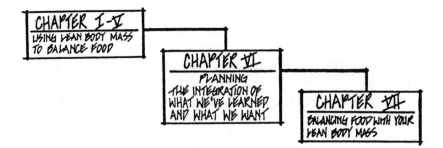

CHAPTER 7

Shopping, Cooking and Eating

"The battle is won or lost at the grocery store."

Overview

The answers to what type of food to eat, what food plan to follow, and how much, when, and how to eat are all in the protein and carbohydrate charts you have constructed. There still remains the hard part. Clients say, "It's easy on paper, but what is really hard is the time shopping, preparing and cooking foods that taste good and support our goals."

Those of us responsible for our family's food know only too well that most of our time can be dominated by food-related activities. The good news: There is a life outside of shopping, cooking, serving food, doing dishes, and planning the next meal.

The number of available cookbooks seems to indicate that our attention is very often on eating and cooking. Perhaps it would be more effective to begin by having our focus on shopping. No one seems to remember that until we buy the food, the cooking and the eating cannot happen. This chapter will develop an approach for convenient, efficient and creative shopping that is outside of our normal thought pattern. This same approach can be adapted to cooking and eating.

The Strategy of Shopping

The majority of us will eat whatever food happens to find its way into the house. So it is true: The battle is won or lost at the grocery store. The shopping list is your battle plan, and the key to your success will be the weekly plan you prepare in advance. It is not wise to go into battle without preparation.

It is a commonly held belief that food, especially the "wrong food," makes us fat and keeps us that way. If we stop for a moment and take an honest look, the real problem might be the person who actually does the shopping.

Initially, we may have food as the enemy, the grocery store as the battle ground, and shopping as the battle; or we may have the kitchen as the battle ground, and eating as the battle. The feeling of winning may be vital to our success at first. Then ultimately, our approach shifts from antagonists to partnership. The grocery store and the restaurant become places we go to obtain vital proteins, fats and carbohydrates to nourish our Lean Body Mass.

I like to picture the grocery store as a giant buffet for shoppers. The similarities between shopping and eating at a buffet are astounding. Imagine we are researchers, and can watch what people buy as they go through the store. After we have observed for a short time, we could predict which foods these people would buy, even before they walked in the store, simply by observing their bodies. After a bit more research, we could predict their energy level throughout the week. We could also predict which families will have a higher incidence of heart problems, arthritis, high blood pressure, and many other chronic illnesses.

Shopping can also be used in a positive and life-enhancing manner, just as food and training can be used to enhance our goals and move us to a position of optimum health and wellness.

Shopping: Your Plan of Attack

The foods we like are listed in the protein and carbohydrate intake charts. The Composition of Foods Table tells us which of our preferred foods have the least fat calories. A weekly meal plan will give us the chance to program which meals will combine protein and carbohydrate, and which meals will keep them separate. Considering that most of these choices have already been made, the shopping list has already been created for us before we sit down to write it out.

Does this process sound familiar? In Chapter One, our Lean Body Mass and activity revealed the calories we use. In chapter three we chose the percentages and the grams of food components from the intake charts, based on our body composition evaluation. We could even say the shopping list is created from the body composition result. The reason this entire process works is because it is all based on a sound physiological fact: your Lean Body Mass.

These steps are to help develope a shopping strategy.

1. Start your week with the first day of your weekend, to allow two days for shopping and preparation. This process will not take the entire two days, and weekends will give you more flexibility and time.

2. Design meals and training for the week in advance.

3. Create your shopping list from the foods you like, and buy only what is on the list.

4. Shop after eating to eliminate impulse buying.

5. Use the outside aisles of the store, as these are the areas most of the foods you will need are located.

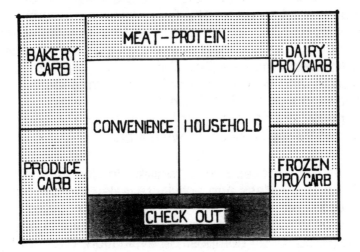

Make shopping a game. Plan your time for shopping, and then time yourself in the store. The shopping list is the key! Ultimately, shopping for the week can be completed in one hour. Anything forgotten can be added to your list for the next time. Consider shopping once for the week, with one more trip at midweek if necessary.

The problem with shopping occurs when we wander through the grocery store, and buy what inspires us. It would be worthwhile to develop a shopping guide with a diagram of the body, and then indicate where each food will go after it is eaten. Protein and carbohydrates would go to the Lean Body Mass, while excess fat and sugar would go to the fat storage areas we all have and know so well. It might be helpful to develop a philosophy of food shopping that is similar to clothes shopping:

Buy only foods that "look good on you!"

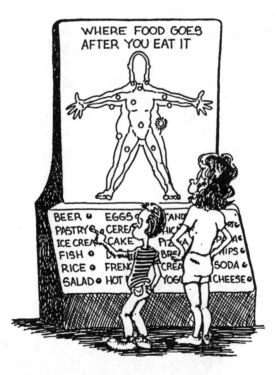

Many people think in terms of one meal, or one day, at a time when shopping or cooking. This is one of the old patterns I invite you to change. The reason we feel locked in, have no time, and are dominated by food-related activities is the one-meal-at-a-time concept. In this situation, food is in charge of you! Wouldn't it be fun to switch roles for awhile? I suggest you be in charge for the next few weeks. If it doesn't work, you will find it very easy to go back to your old system of one meal at a time.

The new possibility is to shop for the entire week in one trip. You will save time in the store, and still be able to select the food that fits your program. The benefit of this strategy is that your shopping will become a model for your entire food program, efficient and lean.

Improving the composition of your body depends on the composition of your food, which further depends on the composition of what is in your shopping cart. It is impossible for us to have an excessive fat content on our body without having a similar composition of fat in our foods. Theoretically, the shopping cart contents could be tested for protein, carbohydrate and fat ratios, because of the similarity between the person's composition, and the composition of the food in the cart.

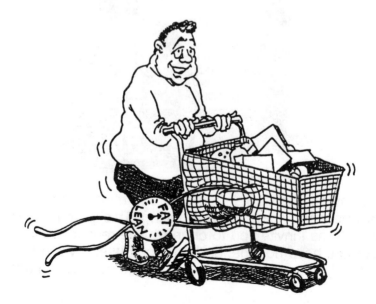

Reducing the fat in foods means altering our grocery shopping. The concern I hear most often is, "Isn't this health food much more expensive?" "Health" food often means different things, depending on who is speaking. When referring to health food, I am referring to protein, fat and carbohydrate foods balanced to match your program; and these are present in the foods you already like.

The Cost of Shopping

Perhaps we should look at the cost of not eating well before examining the cost of shopping. The bottom line is that eating poorly, regardless of how it is done, results in fat. There is an emotional and psychological cost with being over-fat, and with programs that don't work. We also pay a price in decreased health over a period of time. In addition to other costs, we end up paying for medications or diet and reducing plans. Another very real expense is the time spent not improving, when we could be getting better. Compared to the costs mentioned, it would seem that it would be worth any expense for food that worked, and produced the results we wanted.

Although most clients are concerned initially with what might appear to be an increase in food costs, their fears are quickly calmed when they realize that eating more complex carbohydrates and proper amounts of protein results in vast savings. One of the savings occurs when we eliminate much of the expensive packaged and preprocessed foods, and those substances with high fat content, which always increase the costs of our foods.

Now that you know the gram amounts you need each meal, for protein, fat and carbohydrate, review the following tables (Figures 33 - 34, pp. 204 - 205), and consider the "cost" of the food your body requires.

COST OF PROTEIN MEAL - 20 GRAMS

ITEM	AMOUNT/OZ.	FAT/GRAM	COST
Beef - Hot Dogs	6 oz.	41 grams	1.12
Beef - Ground 30% Fat	4 oz.	25 grams	.37
Beef - Ground 15% Fat	3.5 oz.	10 grams	.35
Beef - Rump Roast	4 oz.	36 grams	.48
Beef - T-Bone Steak	5 oz.	47 grams	1.20
Beef - Top Sirloin Steak	5 oz.	44 grams	1.60
Cheese - Cheddar	3 oz.	25 grams	.44
Cheese - 2% Cottage	6 oz.	1 gram	.28
Chicken - Whole Prepared with Skin	2 oz.	2 grams	.20
Chicken - Breasts Prepared without Skin	2 oz.	2 grams	.74
Chicken - Breasts, Boneless, Skinned	2 oz.	2 grams	1.56
Chicken - Breasts, Canned	3 oz.	10 grams	.92
Eggs - Whole	3 eggs	20 grams	.16
Eggs - Whites	6 eggs	0 grams	.32
Fish - Halibut, Fresh	3 oz.	7 grams	.81
Fish - Orange Roughy	3.5 oz.	7 grams	1.20
Fish - Red Snapper	3.5 oz.	.7 grams	.57
Fish - Light Tuna in Oil	3.5 oz.	12 grams	.49
Fish - Light Tuna in Water	3.5 oz.	3 grams	.56
Fish - White Tuna in Water	3.5 oz.	3 grams	.89
Milk - 2%	16 oz.	8 grams	.19
Peanut Butter	3.5 oz.	52 grams	.42
Pork - Bacon	8 oz.	158 grams	.99
Pork - Chops	2.5 oz.	20 grams	.30
Pork - Ham	3 oz.	29 grams	.79
Pork - Ham, Canned	4 oz.	13 grams	1.00
Pork - Ham, Lunch Meat	3 oz.	22 grams	.72
Pork - Ham, Lunch Meat 95% Fat Free	3 oz.	6 grams	.95
Pork - Roast	3 oz.	29 grams	.29
Pork - Sausage	4 oz.	10 grams	.44
Seafood - Crab	4 oz.	2 grams	1.20
Seafood - Shrimp	4 oz.	.8 grams	1.96
Turkey - Canned, White Meat	3.5 oz.	12.2 grams	.70
Turkey - Frozen Dinner	2.5 oz. or 1/2 Dinner	17 grams	.54
Turkey - Lunch Meat 95% Fat Free	3 oz.	5 grams	1.04
Turkey - Whole Fresh, Prepared w/out Skin	2 oz.	2 grams	.36

Figure 33 - Cost of a Protein Meal

COST OF CARBOHYDRATE MEAL - 60 GRAMS

ITEM	AMOUNT/OZ.	FAT/GRAM	COST
Beans - Pinto, Canned	13 oz.	1 gram	.39
Beans - Pinto, Dry	3 oz.	1 gram	.09
Bread - Wheat	4.5 oz.	4.5 grams	.23
Bread - White	4.5 oz.	4.5 grams	.23
Bread - French	4 oz.	2 grams	.12
Cereal - Low Sugar, Boxed	2.5 oz.	2.5 grams	.31
Cereal - Regular Sugar, Boxed	3 oz.	3 grams	.48
Cereal - Oatmeal	3 oz.	.6 grams	.06
Cereal - Instant Oatmeal	3 oz.	.6 grams	.10
Cereal - Instant Oatmeal Flavor Packets	3 oz.	6 grams	.48
Cucumbers	60 oz.	1.2 grams	3.60
Flour	3 oz.	.7 grams	.05
Mushrooms	50 oz.	4 grams	6.00
Nectarines	12.5 oz.	0 grams	1.50
Orange	17.6 oz.	.8 grams	.52
Pasta - Dry Weight	3 oz.	1.4 grams	.14
Pasta - Hamburger Helper	7 oz.	34 grams	1.40
Pasta - Instant Salad	11 oz.	41 grams	3.74
Pasta - Instant Stroganoff	11 oz.	27 grams	2.90
Pasta - Macaroni & Cheese, as packaged	6.5 oz.	1 gram	.46
Pasta - Macaroni & Cheese, as prepared	6.5 oz.	9 grams	.46
Popcorn	3 oz.	4 grams	.08
Popcorn - Microwave	4 oz.	30 grams	.82
Potato - Idaho	10 oz.	.2 grams	.10
Potato - White	10 oz.	.2 grams	.30
Potato - Instant Flakes	2.5 oz.	.4 grams	.22
Potato - Instant Salad	13 oz.	33 grams	4.80
Rice	3 oz.	.3 grams	.08
Rice - Instant	3 oz.	.3 grams	.24
Rice - Instant Pilaf Mix	3 oz.	14grams	.43
Sweet Potatoes - Fresh	8 oz.	.4 grams	.38
Tomatoes - Canned	46 oz.	2 grams	2.30
Tomatoes - Fresh	46 oz.	2 grams	1.80
Yogurt - Vanilla	18 oz.	5.5 grams	.90
Zuchinni Squash - Fresh	60 oz.	1 gram	2.40

Figure 34 - Cost of a Carbohydrate Meal

The Shopping List

In the past I created my grocery list using a method that seems to be common for most of us. I would look in the refrigerator and the cupboard to see what was needed--as if the refrigerator and the cupboard knew. I thought about what was missing, tried to remember what different family members liked, and eventually resorted to the old standby: "I'll wander through the aisles of the store for inspirational ideas from the shelves." The problems I encountered were these:

- Guessing at how much was needed, and usually running out of food midweek.

- Family comments like, "The same old thing again!"

- The family comment, "What's this stuff?", anytime I bought a new food,

It's time for a different approach to the shopping list. The foods that we prefer have already been recorded in our preferred protein and carbohydrate charts. At this point, we let our future shape decide the type and amount of food. The list is written from your weekly meal plan. The weekly meal plan is actually a part of your weekly activity calendar.

Looking at your week in advance is much more than an exercise in saving time. From the standpoint of food, planning the week in advance "creates" an opportunity to include some of our natural eating tendencies, such as skipping meals and fun meals, within the number of meals we will eat that have a balance of proteins and carbohydrates. We can also identify future problem areas, such as not having enough time to buy food, when lunches will have to be prepared ahead of time, and arrangements for food when we have to travel and be away from home.

It is common for most of us to wake up, get ready for work, and be preoccupied with what to do for the day. In this state of mind, food is an afterthought, and the results show in our bodies. The planning approach lets us do exactly the same thing with our food: wake up, get ready for work, and have food be an afterthought. In this case, food is an afterthought for a different reason: that is, it is already planned for and taken care of, in advance!

Because of planning, your food is balanced and supports your weight, shape and goals. Food has now become your partner in your body-shaping program, and it is no longer an adversary.

After a few weeks of meal planning and generating your grocery lists in this manner, you will, at some point, realize that you are literally creating your future body, just as your past has created the present you. The fun part of this program is that each of us gets to be in charge of, and responsible for our progress and future improvement.

From Meal Design to Grocery List

There are many versions of meal-planning ideas. This is merely an example which you may use or redesign to fit your activity and lifestyle more exactly. The purpose of this program is to work with many of the problems we connect with not eating properly. We will consider meals at home and meals away, which includes restaurant food, lunches, deli food, fast food, grocery stores, and eating at a friend's house. If time is spent looking at the week in advance, some major choices can be made. These choices will eliminate surprises and prevent many of the breakdowns in your program which undermine progress.

The procedure for filling out the charts is visually summarized in the following map.

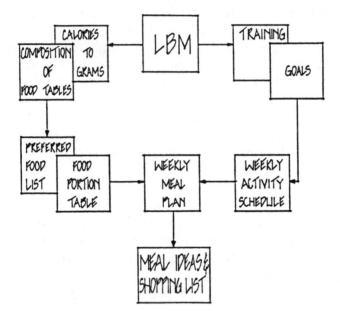

You have already identified your preferred foods and categorized them as proteins, fats, or carbohydrates. The serving size per meal was based on your LBM and activity level. (Chapter 5) The next seven steps lead to a weekly shopping list. Follow the example of a 130 pound working woman. Her goal is to gain 15 pounds of lean mass and lose 35 pounds of fat.

1. Fill out your weekly activity schedule. Include your existing responsibilities and committments. (work, school, meetings, etc.)

2. Specify a time for shopping (1 hour), cooking (3 hours), and training (based on your goals).

3. Choose meal times with the challenge of separating protein and carbohydrates. Identify meals as either protein (P), or carbohydrate (C), or both (P,C).

4. Identify meals you will be responsible for preparing (*), and those meals which will be prepared for you. (restaurants, business lunches, social events, etc.)

5. Determine which meals will be your "fun" meals.

6. Circle all potential problem areas in red. (tight schedule, travel, eating at friends home) This will allow you to plan ahead, in order to prevent breakdowns in your schedule, and keep you on target.

7. Total the protein meals and carbohydrate meals you will be responsible for preparing. This becomes the guide for your shopping list.

The procedure is for filling out the following charts.

HOW TO PLAN YOUR WEEKLY ACTIVITY SCHEDULE TO SUPPORT YOUR GOALS.

LBM Goal: Maintain _____
Gain __15#__

FAT Goal: Maintain _____
Lose __35#__

Current Scores: LBM # __75__   Calories You Use:
FAT # __55__

24 hrs Rest __900__
8-10 hrs Work __180__
1 hr Training __270__
Average Calories Per Day: __1350__

Calories You Will Eat: Day __1080__   Meal __360__
Protein You Will Eat: Day __63__ grams   Meal __21__ grams
Carbohydrates You Will Eat: Day __138__ grams   Meal __46__ grams
Fat You Will Eat: Day __22__ grams   Meal __7__ grams

WEEKLY ACTIVITY SCHEDULE

Time	Sat	Sun	Mon	Tues	Wed	Thurs	Fri
6:00 am			C*MEAL	C*MEAL	P*MEAL	HOTEL	JOY BREAKFAST
7:00 am		P* MEAL				P,C	P,C
8:00 am	C*MEAL					SEMINAR	SEMINAR
9:00 am	LAUNDRY	AEROBICS	WORK	WORK	WORK		
10:00 am	STUDY		P*MEAL	P*MEAL	C*MEAL		
11:00 am	↓P*MEAL					↓	
12:00 pm		BRUNCH – THE CLUB FUN MEAL P,C	LUNCH MEETING P,C MEAL	BUSINESS LUNCH P,C	BUSINESS LUNCH P,C	LUNCH P,C	LUNCH P,C
1:00 pm						SEMINAR	SEMINAR
2:00 pm	BIKE RIDE		WORK	WORK	WORK		
3:00 pm	C*MEAL	SHOPPING & COOKING	↓	↓	↓	↓	
4:00 pm						BREAK WALK!	↓
5:00 pm						SEMINAR	TO AIRPORT
6:00 pm		P*C* MEAL	C*MEAL NIGHT CLASS ↓	P*MEAL	P*C* MEAL	COCKTAILS DINNER	FLIGHT 65
7:00 pm	DINNER DATE			AEROBICS	BUSINESS		P,C MEAL
8:00 pm	P,C MEAL			TRIP PLANE FLIGHT 62	FUN MEAL P,C	CALL FOR SPECIAL LOW/FAT MEAL
9:00 pm			P*MEAL	C*MEAL			
10:00 pm							
11:00 pm							
12:00 am							

Figure 35 - Example Weekly Activity Schedule

HOW TO PLAN YOUR WEEKLY ACTIVITY SCHEDULE TO SUPPORT YOUR GOALS.

LBM Goal: Maintain _____
                      Gain _____
FAT Goal: Maintain _____
                      Lose _____

Current Scores: LBM # _____   Calories You Use: 24 hrs Rest _____
                     FAT # _____   8-10 hrs Work _____
                                                       1 hr Training _____
                                            Average Calories Per Day: _____

Calories You Will Eat: Day _____   Meal _____
Protein You Will Eat: Day _____grams   Meal _____grams
Carbohydrates You Will Eat: Day _____grams   Meal _____grams
Fat You Will Eat: Day _____grams   Meal _____grams

WEEKLY ACTIVITY SCHEDULE							
Time	Sat	Sun	Mon	Tues	Wed	Thurs	Fri
6:00 am							
7:00 am							
8:00 am							
9:00 am							
10:00 am							
11:00 am							
12:00 pm							
1:00 pm							
2:00 pm							
3:00 pm							
4:00 pm							
5:00 pm							
6:00 pm							
7:00 pm							
8:00 pm							
9:00 pm							
10:00 pm							
11:00 pm							
12:00 am							

Figure 36 - Weekly Activity Schedule

EXAMPLE
SHOPPING LIST   # MEALS _9_

SHOPPING STRATEGIES
1. USE A LIST
2. PLAN FOR LEFT-OVERS

PROTEIN

MEAL IDEA	INGREDIENT	AMT	SUPPORTING INGREDIENTS
omelet	eggs	1 doz	salt, pepper, parmesian cheese
	cottage chese	1 quart	
chicken-broiled	chicken breasts.	4 pieces	spices
casserole (rice)			
fish - broiled	check fresh fish	½ lb.	teriyaki, soy sauce.
Tuna salad	Tuna	2 cans	mustard, mayonaise
	mayonaise-lite	1 jar	
	mustard	1 jar	
	celery	1 bunch	
	onions	1 large	
Turkey	sliced turkey-deli	½ lb	bread, mustard, lettuce
Protein shakes	protein powder		
	skim milk	1 quart	
	cocoa	1 box	
Beverages	coffee	1 can	
	diet soda	6-pack	
	sparkling water	1 bottle	

Figure 37 - Example Weekly Shopping List for Protein

SHOPPING LIST PROTEIN	#MEALS _____		SHOPPING STRATEGIES 1. USE A LIST 2. PLAN FOR LEFT-OVERS
MEAL IDEA	INGREDIENT	AMT	SUPPORTING INGREDIENTS

Figure 38 - Weekly Shopping List for Protein

EXAMPLE
SHOPPING LIST   **# MEALS _9_**

CARBOHYDRATE

SHOPPING STRATEGIES
1. USE A LIST
2. PLAN FOR LEFT-OVERS

MEAL IDEA	INGREDIENT	AMT	SUPPORTING INGREDIENTS
oatmeal	oats	1 box	Brown sugar, fruit
	Brown sugar	1 box	
cereal	Bran flakes	1 box	fruit
	skim milk	1 quart	
	nectarines	2	
Rice	Rice	5 lbs.	Raisens
	Raisins	1 lb.	
French toast	Bread	1 loaf	eggs, yogurt, fruit, syrup
	Yogurt	2 cups	
	Bananas	4	
Bagels	Bagels	1 bag (6)	
	Jelly	1 jar	
	margarine	1 tub.	
Pasta (freeze leftovers)	Pasta	2 lbs.	seasonings
- tomatoe sauce	tomatoe sauce	1 jar	
- with veggies	Parmesian cheese	1 jar	
	Broccoli	1 Bunch	
Potatoes	Baking potatoes	4	
Beans	Pinto beans	1 lb.	spices
Jello - low cal	Jello	2 Boxs	fruit
salad	lettuce	1 head	
	tomatoes	4	
	cucumber	1	
	wine vinegar	1 Bottle	
	spices		Basil, tarragon, parsley, curry
other	non-stick cooking spray	1 can	

Figure 39 - Example Weekly Shopping List for Carbohydrates

SHOPPING LIST # MEALS _____			SHOPPING STRATEGIES 1. USE A LIST 2. PLAN FOR LEFT-OVERS
CARBOHYDRATE			
MEAL IDEA	INGREDIENT	AMT	SUPPORTING INGREDIENTS

Figure 40 - Weekly Shopping List for Carbohydrates

It is often a challenge to fit an ideal food and training schedule into our busy week. Only rarely does the ideal schedule actually occur. The objective is to establish the ideal schedule, and then come as close as possible. In any schedule without planning, meals can be random, last minute, and spur-of-the-moment, which leads to eating any food available. Under these circumstances, we turn to convenience foods, which are much higher in fat and more expensive than natural food; and we cannot be certain of the carbohydrate, protein and fat balance. This brings up the immediate concern of time and preparation.

Being able to work with the problem areas, will allow a greater "peace of mind" than any other suggestion regarding your food. The secret here is to identify problem areas that make food preparation inconvenient, and indicate these on your activity calendar. Identifying trouble spots ahead of time will create options, such as preparing food in advance, using leftovers, using a grocery or deli in the area, and other methods to solve the problem before it occurs.

If you have trouble making a choice regarding skipping meals, balancing carbohydrates and proteins, or how many meals to eat correctly, pretend you are designing this meal plan for someone else who is counting on your help. In fact, if you are really interested in having this program work, then plan meals for someone for the week. Find someone you really care about, and set up this person's weekly program in a way that could work for an entire year. This means that if you multiply your weekly program by 52, it would work all year long.

Excess fat in a weekly meal plan could increase body fat by at least 10 pounds in a year. If the weekly plan has too little protein, the person could lose five or more pounds of lean mass by the end of the year. It is valuable to use a plan that will make each week, and each meal, an example we could follow, from the standpoint of proper balance of proteins, fats and carbohydrates.

Some of us will take better care of another person than we will of ourselves. Not only will working with some-one else help to clarify the process, it is also true that there is someone counting on you. The "someone" is your future self, depending upon you to make the com-mitment and then begin improving.

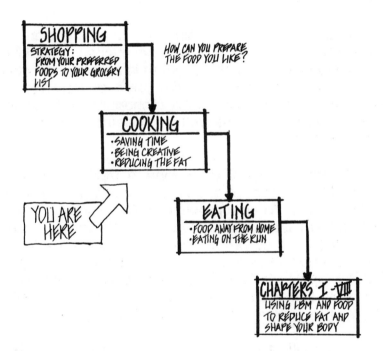

Cooking Concepts

My intention is not to re-invent the information in cookbooks, or alter your standard approach to cooking and eating. People who cook have great ways to prepare food already. People who do not cook have great reasons why it wouldn't fit their schedule.

The challenge occurs when we want to improve our body by reducing fat. Under these circumstances, preparing our own food eventually becomes necessary. If preparing food can be simplified, perhaps we can include homemade food to help speed up the process of losing fat. My main purpose is to stimulate you to be creative, experiment, and use food for the improvement process.

Food Preparation

Just as the process of losing fat and adding lean mass takes time, learning to improve shopping, cooking and eating takes time. This process is an evolution which takes from a few months to a few years, depending upon your involvement. Improving shopping and cooking will mean you spend less time on these activities, as you gain experience.

While the concept of using food to improve is clear, the practical application of actually preparing the food is another matter. When a problem occurs, such as discouragement, it usually has to do with the convenience and method of food preparation. Most people ask for an exact schedule of what they should eat and how they should prepare the food. This is where most diet books, programs, and even experts, get into trouble. They tell you what to eat; and you say, "I don't like that."

I have a different answer to, "What should I eat?" The answer is also a question: "What do you like to eat?" or "How do you like to cook?" There is a great possibility that what you like, and how you cook, may work very well, and would require only a slight alteration.

As you become more familiar with food preparation techniques, you will become the expert at designing the personal food strategy for your body.

Time-Saving Procedures

Perhaps it would be of interest to have the time you spend in kitchen-related activities reduced by 50%. A step that allows this to happen is accumulating the necessary utensils to make food preparation more simple and efficient.

These cookware items are recommended

Blender	Rice steamer	Crock pot
Food processor	Muffin tins	Baking pans
Covered outdoor grill	Griddle	Waffle iron
Assorted pans with lids	Food scale	Pasta pot

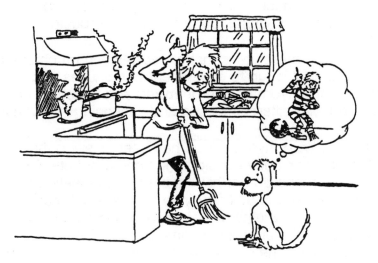

Cooking

The purpose of this section is not to change family recipes, or re-invent thousands of excellent recipes in cookbooks. My intention is to suggest combinations of foods, preparation methods, and flavors, which are convenient. I will attempt to satisfy the rules of food combining, however, there are recipes that combine a small amount of fruit with other foods, primarily carbohydrates. Fruits will not be combined with protein at any time; and, for the most part, fruits that are combined with carbohydrates will be combined during cooking. There will be instances where carbohydrates are combined with protein. While the rules of food combining are valid, there are times for practical purposes, such as, convenience, or flavor we eat certain foods together.

Excessive fats and oils are not used in these cooking recommendations. White sugar, white flour, and some processed foods will be included in the recipes, because these are the most available. It is very easy to substitute whole grain and natural foods for these products.

The main message is that all recipes can be changed if you prefer. It is fun to experiment with sauces and spices. Carbohydrates can be mixed and matched, and prepared with different sauces and seasonings for variety.

Once a carbohydrate food has been chewed the first few times, your body considers it a carbohydrate. Our cells and organs do not have a committee meeting to decide whether the carbohydrate was cereal, bread, rice, or potatoes, or whether it was prepared in a specific way and eaten at the appropriate time of day. Your body does recognize the difference between simple and complex carbohydrates. Nevertheless, carbohydrates are recognized by the body as one of the major food components, and not as specific breakfast, lunch, or dinner foods.

I am aware that our society has rules, standards and beliefs regarding when foods are eaten. As with everything else, we will occasionally adapt the rules to fit our schedules and lifestyles. The one rule to keep in place is to balance the carbohydrates and proteins to our Lean Body Mass and goals. Once the correct amounts of protein and carbohydrates are known, when, how and what to eat is a constant ongoing experiment.

Cooking: The Basics

The major point is: *remove the fat*! When oil is specified in a recipe, use only the oils from vegetables or seeds, and avoid heating them. It is also important to be aware of the fat content in any processed food. Reading the label is a requirement. Looking for ingredients such as; animal fat, lard, and coconut or soybean oil, not only helps you improve your body, in many cases it is life saving. There are volumes of information in well-written books on fat, cholesterol, sodium, and many other problems resulting from poor eating habits. It is time to become your own expert on this subject. You can be assured, that it will be some time before restaurants, grocery stores, and many of the other food providers will alter how they prepare and provide the food.

Substitutions

There are alternatives for all food substances, including fat. You will find many of these ideas in cookbooks on low-fat cooking or eating more natural foods. Learning that recipes in books, or elsewhere, are not sacred is vital. There are no rules you must follow!

What's in the Food?

Not knowing what kind and how many proteins, fats and carbohydrates exist in what you are eating is an invitation for excess fat to come and live on your body. As you may have noticed, fat always establishes residency in the most unwanted spots. There are a number of books to help you learn which foods contain hidden fat calories. One book that includes most grocery items, restaurant foods and "fast foods" is, "*The Complete Book of Food Counts*" by Corinne T. Netzer.

Keep a food scale in your kitchen, in the most obvious and convenient place. Weigh your food as often as possible to be certain the amounts you are eating are correct.

Cooking Multiple Meals

Cooking multiple meals provides extra food to use throughout the week. One possibility is to prepare multiple meals on the weekend when there is more time.

Meals that could be prepared at one time are: skinless turkey on the charcoal grill, a stew in the crock pot, rice in the rice cooker and pasta in a pot on the stove, muffins baking in the oven, along with baked potatoes, and chicken or a casserole. A pan of gravy and a pot steaming vegetables could also be on the stovetop.

All the carbohydrates and proteins you need are ready for the entire week. The foods can also be packaged in individual servings and frozen for future use.

Alternate Meal Concepts for Carbohydrates

There are infinite combinations of tastes and flavors available to us. These concepts are merely "suggestions" and can be used as basic ideas for food preparation. The secret in preparing these foods is simply, use spices for flavor and sauces for variety. The following ideas are for various forms of carbohydrate foods in your diet.

Cereals. Boxed and cooked cereals can easily satisfy our carbohydrate requirements. Be certain, as with all packaged foods, to read the ingredients to determine the fat and sugar content. There are now many whole-grain cereals available. These have less fat than the processed cereals. Cookbooks have many creative recipes for cereals, and what to do with cereal left-overs. Boxed cereals can be a convenient carbohydrate source when traveling or any time you are away from home.

Cereals make a great carbohydrate food anytime of the day. Cold or hot, they can easily be taken to the office or school for snacks. One friend makes extra thick oatmeal, and then cooks the leftovers in thin slices on a griddle for crispy lunches or mid-day snacks. Her children, look for this, and eat it with cinnamon-sugar or jelly for their after-school snack .

 Try placing dry, old-fashioned oatmeal in a bowl. Then cover it with boiling water. Let the water and oats stand three to six minutes, then eat. The oatmeal has a more crunchy texture, which adds variety and a new taste experience.

Grapenuts is a unique dry cereal, in that it doesn't contain oil. It is also a concentrated carbohydrate, which means the volume amount needed to obtain your necessary gram requirement is not large. It is easy to be creative with this cereal by using it as a dry or cooked cereal.

If you prefer, add fruit, sugar, honey or yogurt to the cereal. These are also carbohydrate foods.

Pasta. Many clients think initially that pasta means red sauce and noodles. Pasta is actually the dough, and is usually made from wheat, or other substances, such as corn. Pasta can be in the shape of noodles - thin like spaghetti, thick like lasagna noodles, or various shapes and sizes such as; shells and corkscrews. Pasta is a versatile carbohydrate. Many clients are surprised to learn that pasta noodles can be used in combination with many and seasonings. There are entire books written about this carbohydrate. While pasta contains very little oil, the standard cooking procedures include oil, butter, cheese, and cream sauces. The objective is to enhance the flavor of pasta, and eliminate the fat.

Pasta salad is a convenient and tasty way to obtain carbohydrates. Take the amount of cooked pasta you need and add any vegetables you prefer. (steamed, raw, marinated or plain). Then add spices, and non-fat, dressing. You now have a meal at home or a great lunch anywhere. There are certain non-starchy vegetables, such as cucumbers and celery that contain very few calories. You can increase the volume of your salad without increasing the calorie or carbohydrate amounts.

Another variation with pasta and vegetables, is to combine the vegetables you prefer with your pasta in a non-stick skillet. Blend spices with a small amount of water, and then add this to the skillet mixture. Stir the mixture while it cooks. As the water evaporates and the spices blend into the food, a flavorful meal will be created.

By blending slightly more water, a tablespoon or two of flour, and spices, a gravy is created to cook with the pasta and vegetables. You can interchange any seasoning or spice to create a flavor you prefer. I will remind you that the flavor comes from the food and the spices, not from fat.

Breakfast Pasta. When I say to people, "pasta can be eaten at any time," they nod understandingly until it comes time to actually have pasta for breakfast.

Combine plain pasta in a non-stick skillet with a small amount of water, sugar, cinnamon, and a tablespoon of diet margarine. Stir fry the pasta much in the same way you would prepare oriental vegetables. Some prefer cooking the pasta until crispy for a crunchy texture. Others prefer cooking the pasta until it begins to develop a golden brown color.

As a further stretch of the imagination, it is possible to combine pasta with frozen berries, small amounts of instant vanilla pudding, or molasses, for an incredible carbohydrate dessert.

Another creation with pasta is to make pasta pudding, in much the same manner you would make bread pudding. You can eliminate the fat in the recipe without changing the flavor.

Casseroles: Pasta combined with vegetables and sauces create interesting and diverse casseroles. If you prefer, a protein of your choice can be included to make a complete meal.

Rice. Rice can be used in place of or in combination with pasta in all of the above ideas. Rice can also be used with or without bread in the traditional recipe for bread in stuffing.

Potatoes: Usually we think of potatoes as mashed, baked or scalloped. Potatoes, like most forms of carbohydrates, can be combined in a infinite number of combinations.

It is possible with potatoes, and other carbohydrates, to be so creative with flavors, textures, and combinations that one could be tempted to overlook the protein portion of the meal. Potatoes are low in both carbohydrates and fat. For example, one pound of uncooked potatoes has approximately 75 to 80 grams of carbohydrates, and 4 grams of fat. Potatoes can be substituted in any of the above suggestions, with the exception of the dessert foods.

There are different types of potatoes. A good experiment is to cook three types: red, russet and white, and check out the differences. As long as you are experimenting, don't forget yams and sweet potatoes.

For something different try big chips. Big chips are large slices of potatoes, approximately 1/4 inch thick, baked on the oven rack. You can eat these big chips for snacks, lunches or mix them with other carbohydrate foods.

For a special treat of texture and taste, combine pasta and mashed potatoes with non-fat gravy. They can also be fried in a non-stick skillet for an crispier combination.

Baked Potatoes. Baked Potatoes are a great source of carbohydrates any time. They are easily packed for lunches or travel food and can be combined with an unlimited number of vegetables, spices and flavors. There is always a place for potatoes to be combined with vegetables, casseroles, pancakes, bread batters and a variety of other foods.

Sauces and Gravy: Because many carbohydrates are flavored by the food or seasoning with which it is prepared, sauces and gravies are the perfect combination. They also add moisture, to an otherwise dry carbohydrate. Once the concept of preparing a sauce or gravy without fat is accepted, the only limits to the flavor you create is your own imagination. If there is one rule regarding cooking it should be, "Experiment with different flavors and foods." This will keep the foods interesting, tasty, and eliminate the boredom that comes from eating the same food over and over.

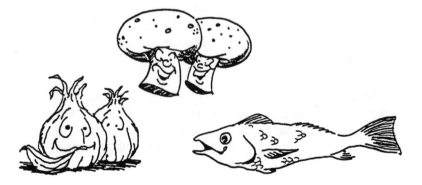

Soups and Stews. Homemade soups and stews can include any number, and variety of carbohydrates; rice, potatoes, pasta or vegetables. Cookbooks have abundant recipes for soups and stews. My only words of caution are that the oil and fats recommended in the recipes are certainly not necessary in the amounts given, and in most cases can be totally eliminated.

Beans. Bean recipes and ideas are abundant in cookbooks. The main suggestion is to avoid oil and lard which are commonly added to this food. Fat and oil are not necessary for cooking or flavor. Beans, like potatoes, are a great nonfat carbohydrate.

Breads, Biscuits, Pancakes and Waffles. Don't avoid them! The bread is not the problem, it is the fat disguised as peanut butter, mayonnaise, and butter, that goes on the bread. Bread by itself contains very little fat. It can be eaten plain, toasted, with salad, steamed vegetables, jellies and dips, or used as croutons.

The main objective with bread is to weigh it before you toast or eat it. You will soon get a sense of the amount that satisfies your carbohydrate requirement. Bread puddings and French toast are just two ideas for excellent and highly available carbohydrate.

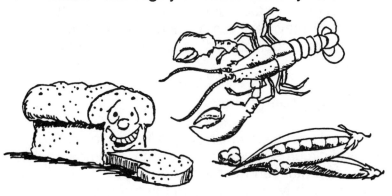

Vegetables. There are two kinds of vegetables, starchy and non-starchy. Starchy vegetables are: peas, corn, and squash. They can be steamed, baked, marinated or added to and combined with other carbohydrate foods in a variety of ways. Non-Starchy vegetables are: cucumbers, lettuce, sprouts, and peppers. They are primarily used for bulk and texture in recipes.

Carbohydrates make up the bulk of your food each meal and each day. In their natural form, they contain very little fat and the necessary vitamins, minerals and enzymes to help your body processes. The natural forms of these foods are best. Start with simple preparation methods, until the concepts are mastered.

Commercial Food

Food prepared commercially includes pizza, TV dinners, desserts, treats, snacks, boxed and packaged cereals, and those foods that we heat and eat. These foods can work for us, if they are considered a carbohydrate or a protein food, and their fat content fits within our goals for each meal. Read the labels and use common sense about the fat content. When you want to celebrate and feel, "You deserve a break today," binge on low-fat treats that will not add as many fat calories per bite. In other words, one bite of a low-fat treat may have less than a gram of fat, but one bite of a very rich dessert or snack may have ten or more grams of fat, and require up to one hour of training to remove that fat from your body.

Food Away From Home

The basic concept which prepares you for eating, under any circumstances, in any place, is simply to think in terms of protein and carbohydrates for your body, and the goals you have set. Although the types of protein and carbohydrate foods change depending on the situation, the grams of protein, determined by your LBM will be the same.

Restaurants

Eating in restaurants takes courage! Ordering the foods you want, and the way you want them prepared, is a great test of your commitment. One question that will prepare you for ordering restaurant food is to consider: "Who is paying the bill?" You might also remember who is working to improve body composition, eating carefully at home, shopping with care to balance protein and carbohydrates, and increasing the quality of a training program. There is a good chance the answer to this question is not the cook, the owner, waiter or waitress. You are the one responsible for your improvement program. It is absolutely essential that you take responsibility for ordering the restaurant food that supports your program.

If the food cannot or will not be prepared as you ask, and you know this ahead of time, be prepared to bring food from home. As you prepare more of your food at home in a manner which restaurants call dry, meaning no oil, you will recognize how it looks, and also become aware of the non-greasy taste. After a certain point, oily food will not be acceptable to you. The following tips can be helpful when eating in restaurants:

1. Ask if food can be prepared without oil or fat. Some methods include baking, charbroiling, poaching and steaming. If calling ahead is not possible, there are other alternatives.

 a. Learn ahead of time whether this particular restaurant would have carbohydrates that will support your program. Or perhaps their preparation of protein would be better for you. For example, a restaurant may be willing to cook your fish or chicken on a charcoal grill, and have only french fries or vegetables sauteed in butter, for your side dish. In this case, you would make other arrangements for the carbohydrate portion of your meal. Some restaurants will have baked potatoes or rice, which would support the carbohydrate portion of your food program and will be unwilling to prepare the protein without oil or a creamy sauce. You will learn creativity as you deal with restaurants.

b. You will find that most salad dressings contain oil. Ask for low-fat ddressing, such as; vinegar or lemon wedges.

c. When discussing food with your waiter or waitress, begin by explaining that because of a medical problem or doctor's orders, you are on a restricted diet, and cannot have foods with oil or any form of grease.

These suggestions help to support you in achieving your goals, while enjoying meals out with family and friends.

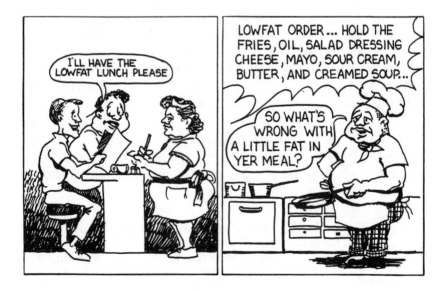

Buffets and Brunches

The vast display of food at a Sunday brunch is over-whelming. Not often do we have the opportunity to stand in one spot and see salads, proteins, carbohydrates and desserts in multiple combinations at the same time. It is not fair for the untrained person to be placed in this situation. There is a way to learn from this experience, which is designed to appeal to, and benefit, only your eyes and mouth. The following is your game plan:

1. Do not play "follow the leader" with anyone else.

2. Eat fruit first! Have whatever plain fruit you prefer, avoid fruit salads, and wait 20 minutes before eating the next type of food.

3. Have carbohydrates next. There are many forms of bread, rice and potato. This does not include noodle salads with mayonnaise, fruit or vegetable salads with oil and/or mayonnaise, and pastries.

4. Eat as much of these carbohydrates as you prefer, and wait 20 minutes before the protein portion of your meal.

5. Have your protein last, or with salad if you prefer.

6. Notice that we have avoided the greasy salads, and have separated fruits, carbohydrates and proteins. After the protein portion of your meal, be aware of how much food you have actually eaten and how you feel. In most cases, by this time you will feel comfortable and not bloated.

At this point, you have a choice. If you miss that over-full feeling which makes the meal complete, you can have either a large helping of fruit or a large dessert. I suspect, in most cases, the over full feeling will be the same. This is only a suggestion. Unless you experiment, you will not know which foods, and which order of eating these foods, works best for you.

Eating on the Run

When you are traveling and it is time for food, there are options other than fast food restaurants. Most of us don't think of grocery stores. Grocery stores have food that is more economical and which will support your program for improving body composition. Rather than thinking in terms of eating and food, remember the basic concepts for supporting your LBM, and think in terms of, proteins and carbohydrates.

QUICK GROCERY STORE FOOD

Protein:	**Carbohydrates:**
canned fish	bread and rolls,
prepackaged turkey	cereals
deli sliced chicken	crackers
sliced turkey breast	Vegetables
low-fat cottage cheese	fruit

Delis and Cafeterias. Major rule: Consider the fat content of the foods. One thing to remember about deli and cafeteria foods is that the pasta and other non-lettuce salads have a high oil content. This is good for taste, and not so good for your body composition.

When eating in delis, select the more lean meats with bread, rolls and bagels. Butter, mayonnaise, cheese and cream cheeses are standard in all sandwiches, and are fat foods.

Fast Foods. We have already mentioned the excellent resource, *The Complete Book of Food Counts* by Corinne T. Netser. The rest is easy. Look up what you like to order in your guide, add the fat grams per meal, and compare this to your maximum amount of fat intake per meal. It takes approximately an hour of constant training at your fat-burning heart rate to use the extra fat you can consume in a few minutes. The sad part is, you may not even know you have eaten the fat.

Doesn't it make more sense to avoid hidden fat, and enjoy a dessert or treat that fits into your food program for the day? If you do not avoid hidden fat, you could be training one hour a day just to use the extra fat you have eaten, without making a reduction in the amount of fat stored on your body. I am not saying you should avoid fast foods. I am simply reminding you to look up the food, be aware of the fat content, and make your choice accordingly.

Airlines, Hospitals, Schools. Anytime food is prepared in large quantities, I advise people to be cautious. Institutional cooking is generally high in fat. Ask specifically how foods have been prepared. Check to see if low-fat meals are available. Voice your concerns to someone who would be able to institute a change. (owner, administrater, chef, etc.) Most airlines will provide a low-fat meal if requested 24 hours in advance. See if this can be arranged when you make your flight reservation. An awareness of the fat in our diets, can change the way foods are prepared.

Basic Principles

The concept I am about to explain applies to more than just food. We have a tendency to think that, when we eat an excess on one day, we can eat less the next two or three days to make up for it. There are many versions of this philosophy. For example, if we undereat or skip meals, we "know" the body will go on performing normally, and we can always grab a snack later on. It is time for you to know the truth.

Your body has no concept of the past, what you did yesterday or last night, and no concept of the future. In other words, your Lean Mass has no idea that you intend to make up for eating incorrectly today by eating properly tomorrow or the next day. It responds instantly, and in harmony with your food program and your activity. When your body needs more protein, carbohydrates or energy, for performance, it either gets the supply that is required, from the fuel you provide, from your muscle or it will not perform optimally.

If your meal is balanced at 60% carbohydrates, 20% protein and 20% fat, you eat the correct number of calories to support your goal, and you eat this meal three times per day for one year, you will see a dramatic improvement in your body by the end of 365 days.

If your meals are low in protein, 365 days later your muscle mass would be significantly less. The same concept holds true for fat. Perhaps the Lean Body Mass is actually a model for us in terms of how we need to take care of ourselves, and approach every part of every day.

The concept of eating, as a tool you can use in your improvement program, will serve you well in this age and culture of fast pace and convenience foods. It is impor

tant to keep in mind, from the standpoint of responsibility, that the composition of the food in the shopping
cart, the food you cook, and the food you eat *becomes*
your body composition.

Wrapping Up

One of the messages in Chapters Four through
Seven is that "any level of body composition you choose
is available to you within your lifestyle!" What you want, in
terms of body composition, is not impossible or withheld
from you because of age, sex, occupation, or genetics.
What actually limits people are their actions, and not
doing what they know must be done. It is not people's
minds that tell them whether their program is working or
not; it is their body composition evaluation. People's
minds, and what they believe, actually create the limits
they place on themselves.

The limits and beliefs we impose on ourselves are
very similar to the belief that aerodynamically, and from
an engineering standpoint, bumblebees cannot fly. The
bee community has given human belief systems very little credibility, having found, through their own research,
that flying is far more efficient than walking from flower to
flower. I suggest you use the same approach that bees
use, and at least question your beliefs, your history and
the belief systems of other humans. Conduct your own
research with food, training and body composition. You
may find the changes you have always wanted happen
with less effort, than you could have possibly imagined.

Many people have preceded you in improving their
body composition and altering weight and shape, changes which were previously thought impossible. A great
body is not a lifetime guarantee; and it doesn't last
without proper food and training! A not-so-great body is
not a lifetime sentence; and it also doesn't last with
proper food and training!

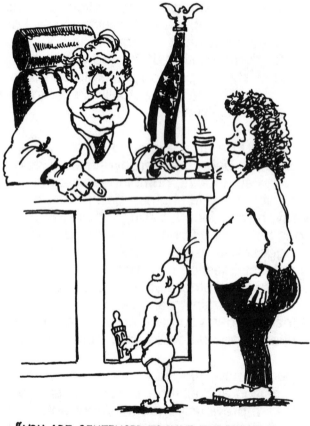

"YOU ARE SENTENCED TO HAVE THE SHAPE OF ALL WOMEN ON YOUR MOTHERS SIDE OF THE FAMILY..... FOR LIFE!!"

CHAPTER 8

Synchrony: Making it Work From Concept to Results

"Everything necessary to create your future body is available today. Your part is to rearrange what's available into a recipe that works within your lifestyle, and is based on your Lean Body Mass."

A New Viewpoint.

When you look at your body from the standpoint of Lean Body Mass and muscle, there are suddenly new opportunities for improvement. This new perspective lets the same old food and same old training become new and alive, and they become your partners for improvement, rather than your adversaries. You no longer have to avoid food in order to improve. Now, food is something you *include* in order to improve. Training shifts from a "have to do," to something you actually play at and experiment with, in order to design and sculpt your body.

An Invitation

From your body's perspective, you have never changed suddenly. You grew up, grew older, and got "out of shape" over a period of time, and now you are invited to grow better from this moment on. Keep in mind that your body doesn't understand "slow" or "fast." It works perfectly, according to your Lean Mass, food and activity. Your Lean Body Mass is doing all it can with the food and activity you are supplying.

Permission

Consider this chapter a certificate which gives you full permission to experiment and be creative with your training and food. How creative can you be? Look at how creative you can be in order to avoid a responsibility or commitment. Do not discount or underestimate your creativity. Most of us use our creative side to find quick ways to control weight, and skip training sessions. We keep coming up with new ways to improve overnight.

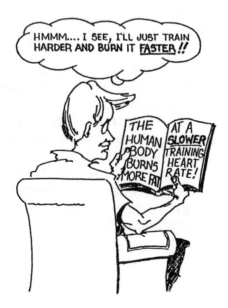

These methods don't work. They are all designed to "beat the system." What system? The one that says there are 3,600 calories in one pound of fat, and our Lean Body Mass needs to use 3,600 calories to eliminate one pound of fat. Rather than trying to outsmart our body, why not use our creativity to work with the LBM for an individualized, accurate improvement program?

The Truth

The body composition evaluation is an interesting way of finding out "the truth." The evaluation is like looking in an absolutely honest mirror, and it gives your Lean Body Mass a chance to tell you how well you have been taking care of yourself.

The body composition evaluation reveals much more than pounds and percentages. It is an objective report that states, "You improved," or "You did not improve." The results are based on your last few weeks, or months, of food and training! Your improvement, or lack of improvement, is okay, and not right, wrong, good or bad. It is simply what happened. You then have the opportunity to commit to your next two-to-four week training and food program, and check again with the next body composition evaluation.

You don't have to be "perfect" before starting an improvement program. The minute you begin to improve, before it is visible, you feel more alive and attractive. There are many effective methods and courses to improve your thought process. There are only a few technologies accurately designed to improve your body for life. The body composition evaluation can truly become a partner in helping to improve your Lean Body Mass.

Your Guarantee

Wouldn't it be exciting to create an environment or structure that would absolutely guarantee the results you want in the area of Lean Body Mass, reducing fat and improving your shape? A foundation is necessary before we can create the structure to make it all happen.

The standard concern is being able to start and continue any program. In setting up our structure for success, there must be a starting point. We could say the beginning of starting, or what actually precedes starting, is wanting. Most of us want a better body. How badly we want a better body will drive us to achieving a specific result.

Getting the Results You Want

Having the body you want cannot be just another casual request. Casual does not guarantee success. The person who is successful can create a want so big, it is an absolute hunger. It becomes a passionate desire accompained by a willingness to discover, and work through any barriers that have stopped your improvement programs in the past.

Let's discuss wants from another perspective, and see if this is a commitment you want to make. You might say you "want" to train and you "want" a better body, but never get around to training. The unspoken statement is: You want the comfort and convenience of not training more than the inconvenience of exercise.

The solution to this problem is creating a "want" so big, that training is included and happens automatically. For example, we could create reasons for developing your new body that are truly great, such as becoming an example for your friends and family, and being available for activities with your grandchildren. Once the "big want" is established, which requires a healthy, energetic body, training might be the best way to accomplish your goal. As you focus on the larger picture, training becomes an automatic process. Training for the sake of big biceps, slender thighs and a flat stomach is not incentive enough to keep you motivated for very long.

At this point, I would review how much you would be willing to invest in time and effort in order to accomplish the result. The human trait is to use weight loss clinics, fad diet plans, doctors, pills and programs for a quick change. The natural law and the way the body works requires proper training and food, over a period of time. I am not asking what your mind, your schedule or your comfort would prefer. I am asking what you really *want*.

After you decide what you want, a series of tests occurs. You are tested in the following ways. When it is time for a training program, your body would rather rest, your mind would prefer a TV break, your ear would enjoy the telephone, your mouth wouldn't mind a snack, and you begin thinking about how little sleep you had the night before. This is called "being human," and you are doing what we all do. We lump all of the preferences and wants of our little individual parts together, and we forget our giant commitment to be lean.

Our objective here is to become aware that our smaller, more immediate, wants are always present, and shouldn't be confused and run together to outnumber our bigger purpose. All your conscious mind knows is that you have seven little wants for immediate gratification and one big want for your long-term goal. Unfortunately, your mind doesn't distinguish objectives, like little and big, and so the final score is seven to one. Broken down, that is seven wants that do not include training, and one want that will make a difference for you and your body. The rest is your choice.

As an illustration that wanting can be separated from having and an example of how children understand this concept so much better than we grownups, I have a story concerning one of my favorite people. When Kendra Lee was five, we would stand in front of the huge grocery store candy display, and talk about wanting each of the candies. We talked about our mouth wanting candy, and our bodies not wanting the candy because we didn't want to be fat. She would explain to me, "It is OK not to have the candy, because just wanting the candy is enough."

What Happens When You Stop?

The kind of "wanting a better body" I'm describing was made clear to me in a discussion with an overweight friend who said, "I've got it! I know what I really want for my body." She explained, "I want to look so good that when I walk into a room, it knocks people out!" "You mean, fall over?" I asked. She said, "I don't want anyone to be hurt, but I want them to gasp . . . just a little!"

Have you ever felt you, or someone else, were wrong for stopping a food or training program? It never occurs to us that stopping is simply not continuing. Stopping is not the issue; it is how long you wait before starting again that is the problem. Stopping is a part of any process. What you do with stopping makes the difference.

I recently listened to an accomplished runner, talk with a beginner, who was complaining about her lack of consistency in her training program. The seasoned runner answered, "I completely understand and sympathize with you. I always stop my program." "You do?" asked the novice. "Yes," answered the veteran runner, "then I sleep, and start again the next day."

There is an opportunity here to give yourself a break. Don't feel wrong for stopping; just sleep and start again each day. When you think about it, isn't that what we do anyway: stop, go to sleep and wake up the next day to start again? So, after starting, you get to continue. The definition of continuing is lots of "starting overs" linked together closely.

Many people wait until Monday to start their food and training program. When a breakdown happens on Tuesday, the unwritten and unspoken rule is that the person does whatever he or she wants, until the following Monday when it is time to start again. The best way to remedy this situation is to put a calendar on the refrigerator or bathroom mirror, and substitute the word "Monday" for each day of the week.

The Structure for Success

The next question is, "How will you set up your training, so you must succeed?" Said another way, how do you box yourself in, so there is no way to fail?

The first step is to create your vision on the basis of what you want! The next step is planning or designing your week and day, as described in Chapters Six and Seven. And the third step, before discussing the actual structure, is in the form of a question that needs to be honestly answered before you proceed: "What would be the problem with having the body, lean mass, shape and energy level you have always wanted?"

Although this appears to be an unusual question, it seems that many of us would not want to accomplish our goal, because we might look too good. The following are only a few answers I have received in response to the above question:

- I'd have to buy all new clothes.

- All my friends are fat, and they would be jealous.

- My spouse would think I was having an affair.

- I wouldn't know what to say and how to act.

Each of us can creatively undermine any success plan, if we feel that looking better is a problem. "Looking better" to set an example for your friend or family is a way of using your creativity to insure your success, rather than to undermine your progress. I know you are creative enough to establish your own success plan.

It might be helpful to look at what successful people do to establish success structures, and possibly apply these principles to our training and food programs. Even the most successful people would be totally ineffective without a structure or manager. A structure could mean your office, job, certain hours, people you answer to, and the ideas and data you use to accomplish results. A manager might possibly be a person, such as a coach or trainer, doctor, or friend. Your schedule, or appointment book, can also support your success.

The best example of a structure that works, in spite of how we feel, is school. The school schedule is set up ahead of time. We complain, and yet we get results, because we are automatically involved in the process. People who are effective have specific projects to accomplish in a day, and specific intervals between projects. Random action seldom works in business or personal settings; yet, it is what we do most easily. When it comes to our training program, the mood is frequently, "I'll see what the scale says this morning, or how tight my clothes are, and then I'll train."

People who want accomplishment in any area monitor their results by establishing goals, daily or week-ly meetings with their own group, or attend larger meet-ings to learn more about their particular interests. They work with employees, partners and employers in a way that benefits themselves and their business. There is definitely a plan, so they are actually managed by what they want to create.

Winning: A Strategy

People have used one or more of these systems, with excellent results. I personally have needed to work with all of them. My own commitment to be at my optimum physically is great, and so is my ability to get out of that commitment. What has worked, and continues to be ef-fective for me, is to set up a system of support ahead of time, so I cannot help but accomplish the goal or project. It is interesting to note the same system works with food.

1. Establish who you are in the process of becoming.

2. Be realistic about your goals.

3. Be realistic about time.

4. Create a schedule.

5. Keep a journal.

6. Choose your monitoring system.

7. Develop and use your personal support system.

Establish who you are in the process of becoming.

A statement of who you are becoming should be short and positive. One example might be:

> "I am a vibrant and alive woman with 107 pounds of Lean Body Mass. I have the determination, commitment and desire to have my optimum Lean Body Mass of 110 pounds and reduce my body fat 12 pounds, 14 months from today (date).

This type of list will require courage. When you make a bold statement, ahead of the time, you are creating what will occur. The first concern is usually, "I don't know if I can really accomplish this". The concern is valid, and you make the statement anyway! Not being this clear, passionate and involved in your weight and shape has resulted in your present condition. Why not begin with a declaration of who you really are, according to your Lean Body Mass? The exciting part is stating your declaration to others, and having them support you. Setting up your support structure with great detail guarantees your success.

Be realistic about your goals.

Review what you have learned in Chapters One, Two and Three regarding your muscle mass and present amount of fat. Chapter Four, explains your rate of change for adding lean mass and reducing fat.

Take everything into consideration, including the length of time you have been inactive, how long your body has been at its present composition, and allow yourself time to change. (Your rate of change will match your body, time, schedule and training.) Your improvement will not proceed according to the wild claims you see advertised in magazines and on television.

Be realistic about time.

If you add the work hours, sleeping time and eating time, there are a number of hours left over each day, and even more on weekends. Next, list your commitments-- meetings, family, social events--and determine how much time is left. The choice is to commit these hours to being a participant, or to being a spectator. (The time frame for changing your body is discussed in more detail in the chapter on training.)

The challenge here is to determine if the words during spectator time are given mostly to complaints, or to the type of conversation that generates action. Once you have made the choice to train, the amount of time you will have for this activity will almost create itself, without interfering with your other scheduled events.

Create a schedule.

A schedule is of vital importance to having your system work. This could be a monthly calendar, a day planner or any means of allowing you to schedule your time in "advance." Here is the key! You do the planning! Do not wait to see if you will have time to fit in training--plan the training in advance.

One of the better ways to plan training is to start with a calendar at the beginning of the month, and consider Saturday and Sunday as training days, instead of rest days. Your body does not understand weekends. After creating your plan, box yourself in, so there is no escape. We all tend to plan our training for the "next day, maybe, if we get our other projects done, if there is time, and if we are in the mood." The larger commitment for your body is to have your training set up in advance.

Keep a journal

Your journal is another key factor to guarantee your success. The journal becomes your manager, when you establish your training plan in advance. It becomes your memory in keeping track of what you have done, your improvements, and your progress, with your shape, weight, and performance goals.

I will recommend one type for you, initially. This particular system, called the Franklin Day Planner, has a three-cassette series of instructions regarding the use of your day planning system. The instructions create the same type of planning you have been using to design your food and training. Also, your journal provides a planning calendar up to five years in advance, so you can plan for your future body.

Choose your monitoring system

If the journal could be considered your memory, the body composition evaluation, as a monitoring system, is definitely your conscience.

In most areas, we want absolute truth. For example, we have speedometers on our cars, gas and oil gauges to prevent problems, blood pressure and cholesterol tests as monitoring systems of our cardiovascular system, and infinite other ways of finding out the truth, including thermometers, clocks and checkbooks. It seems only logical that we monitor the most precious piece of equipment we have, and the one that will be vastly more important to us in the years to come, our Lean Body Mass.

Develop and use your personal support system

Support systems include people, places to train, and equipment. How you actually interact with your support system in order to lock in your success, is crucial.

Keep in mind, for this discussion, that you have a major commitment to improve your body, using training and food. In order to work with these systems over the years, I was, and still am, on the receiving end of some very frank discussions from the people who support me. I, like you, have the creative ability to get out of my commitments. It took some time to learn to use my creativity and lock myself into commitments for my own good.

When your goal is set, you will be ready to create your own support. Depending upon your activity, your support team could include family, friends, coaches, advisors or health care professionals. To succeed, you will need to know that how "support" looks and feels is different from what you might expect.

You are interested in support, not sympathy. This support is the same as that received when you asked Mom how to spell a word, and she said, "Look it up in the dictionary." The traffic patrolman uses the same support system in reminding us not to speed, and teachers support us with an appropriate grade when we haven't studied. We usually hear, "The teacher gave me a bad grade." Occasionally, a responsible person will say, "I didn't study, so the teacher gave me the grade I deserved." The grade is support in terms of a reminder, and the comments and support from the people on the team should be much like the body composition evaluation: truthful, honest, and hold us to our commitment.

People that support you will do whatever is necessary for you to win. They will inspire you; they will be direct; they will challenge, and even intimidate, you, if that's what it takes to help you accomplish what you want.

Many of us are not ready to work with, and actually face, what is in the way of our improvement. To succeed, it is important to realize no one does this alone. Your support structure must include experts, beginners, partners and everyone else in your environment. You also must ask for their support to work with you on accomplishing your goals. The key regarding support is: While people are supporting you to reach your goals, find other people you can, in turn, support to achieve their goals for weight and shape.

Soon you will realize it is not the people supporting you, it is you becoming an example and supporting others, that will continue your growth and keep you motivated. This is, indeed, *The Lean Body Promise.*

Wrapping Up

The Lean Body Promise provides all the information to create your future body. Information or knowledge alone does not produce results. Action produces results. What gets us started and keeps us in "action", in spite of constant interruptions, is a focus on the bigger picture.

The vision you have for your life is the bigger picture. What keeps you involved is when your vision is personal, dynamic and important enough to let you learn from the always present blocks and barriers.

My vision for *The Lean Body Promise* is to alter forever the relationship people have with their food, activity and body as demonstration that health, weight, shape, vitality and performance are a choice.

What keeps me involved, and keeps this vision expanding are the the results I see with others. Our lean mass is us and is what links us to each other and our environment. The way we acknowledge, nurture and develop our physical potential reflects the way we nurture and develop our world.

In a unique way, each of us is a model for the future. To know the future is a choice we make today inspires a daily commitment to our future self.

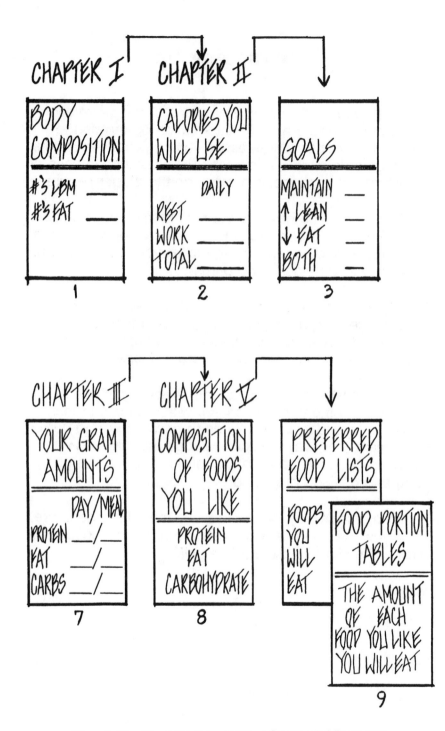

Figure 41 - Final Update of Your Goals and Program

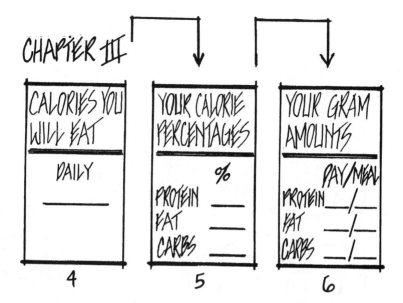

CHAPTER III

CALORIES YOU WILL EAT	YOUR CALORIE PERCENTAGES	YOUR GRAM AMOUNTS

DAILY

PERCENTAGES %

PROTEIN ____
FAT ____
CARBS ____

AMOUNTS DAY/MEAL

PROTEIN ____/____
FAT ____/____
CARBS ____/____

4   5   6

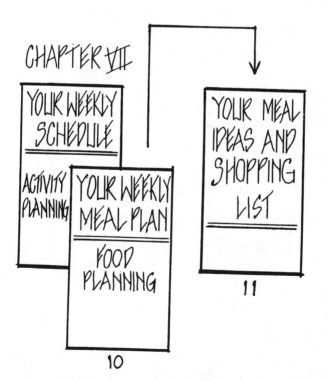

CHAPTER VII

YOUR WEEKLY SCHEDULE

ACTIVITY PLANNING

YOUR WEEKLY MEAL PLAN

FOOD PLANNING

YOUR MEAL IDEAS AND SHOPPING LIST

10   11

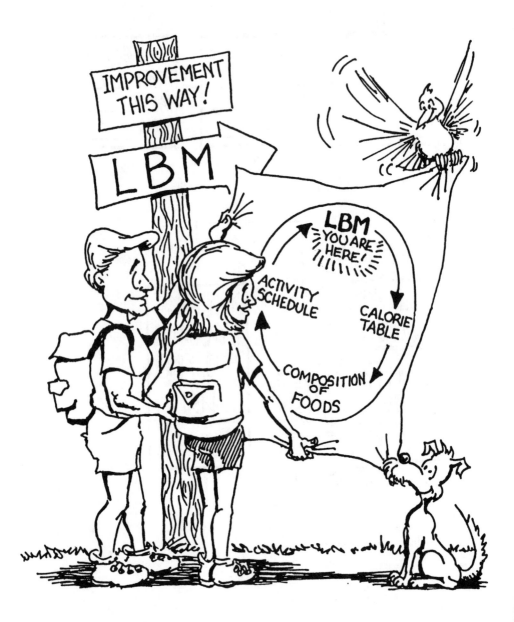

Appendix 1

Composition of Foods Table

Are the foods you like helping you improve? One answer is to look in a "food dictionary" called The Composition of Foods Table. The table will provide a breakdown of each food into its gram amount for each major food component. The symbol in the left margin is an instant reference regarding the protein, fat and carbohydrate classification of the food.

Using the new classification system to identify fat content in foods will simplify your food choices, eliminate confusion, and help you recognize foods that stand in the way of your progress. See Chapter Five for a complete explanation and step by step format to use the food table. The symbols and their classifications are:

+	yellow	protein
+/-	orange	protein high in fat
-	red	fat
*/-	purple	carbohydrate high in fat
*	blue	carbohydrate

Use the blank spaces to add foods & your food portions.
NOTE: tr. is less than or equal to .09 gram

Standard Portion - 100 grams or 3 1/2 ounces

	food	cal	pro gms	fat gms	carb gms
+	Abalone - raw	98	18.7	0.5	3.4
+	Albacore - raw	177	25.3	7.6	0.0
-	Almonds - dried	598	18.6	54.2	19.5
-	Anchovy	176	19.2	10.3	0.3
	Apples				
*	raw	58	0.2	0.6	14.5
*	dehydr., uncooked	353	1.4	2.0	92.1
*	dehydr., cooked	76	0.2	0.3	19.6
*	Apple Butter	186	0.4	0.8	46.8
*	Apple Juice - dilluted	47	0.1	tr.	11.9
	Applesauce				
*	canned - unsweetened	41	0.2	0.2	10.8
*	canned - sweetened	91	0.2	0.1	23.8
	Apricots				
*	raw	51	1.0	0.2	12.8
*	canned, heavy syrup	86	0.6	0.1	22.0
*	dehydr., uncooked	332	5.6	1.0	84.6
*	dehydr., cooked	119	1.3	0.2	30.5
*	Apricot Nectar - dilluted	57	0.3	0.1	14.6
	Artichokes				
*	raw	9	2.9	0.2	10.6
*	boiled/steamed	8	2.9	0.2	10.6
	Asparagus				
*	raw	26	2.5	0.2	5.0
*	boiled/steamed	26	2.5	0.2	5.0
-	Avacados - raw	167	2.1	16.4	6.3
	Baby Food Cereal				
*	mixed	368	15.2	2.9	70.6
*	oatmeal	375	16.5	5.5	66.0
*	rice	371	6.6	1.6	80.0
	Baby Food Desserts				
*	banana tapocia	84	0.4	0.2	21.6
*	custard pudding	100	2.3	1.8	18.6
*	fruit pudding	96	1.2	0.9	21.6
*	fruit	84	0.3	0.3	21.5

Standard Portion - 100 grams (3 1/2 ounces)

	food	cal	pro gms	fat gms	carb gms
	Baby Food Dinners				
*	beef noodle	48	2.8	1.1	8.8
*	chicken noodle	49	2.1	1.3	7.2
*	chicken vegetable, cereal	64	2.1	1.4	7.7
*	ham vegetable, split pea	80	4.0	2.1	11.2
*	macaroni, tomato, meat	67	2.6	2.0	9.6
-	Bacon - cooked	611	60.4	52.9	3.2
*	Bamboo Shoots - raw	27	2.6	0.3	5.3
*	Bananas - raw	85	1.1	0.2	22.2
*	Barley - light	349	8.2	1.0	78.8
+	Bass - raw	93	19.2	1.2	0.0
	Beans				
*	white, raw, dry	340	22.3	1.6	61.3
*	white, cooked	118	7.8	0.6	21.2
*	red, raw, dry	343	22.5	1.5	61.9
	Beef				
	Prime Grade				
	(54% lean - 46% fat)	428	13.6	41.0	0.0
	Choice Grade				
-	(60% lean - 40% fat)	379	14.9	35.0	0.0
	Good Grade				
-	(66% lean - 34% fat)	323	16.5	28.0	0.0
	Standard Grade				
-	(73% lean - 27% fat)	266	18.0	21.0	0.0
	Corned Beef				
-	cooked - medium fat	372	22.9	30.4	0.0
-	canned - fat	263	23.5	18.0	0.0
+/-	med. fat	216	25.3	12.0	0.0
+	lean	185	26.4	8.0	0.0
	Hamburber				
	ground beef - lean				
+/-	raw	179	20.7	10.0	0.0
+/-	cooked	219	27.4	11.3	0.0
	regular ground				
-	raw	268	17.9	21.2	0.0
-	cooked	286	24.2	20.3	0.0

Standard Portion - 100 grams (3 1/2 ounces)

	food	cal	pro gms	fat gms	carb gms
	Porter House Steak				
	choice grade				
-	raw (63%lean - 37% fat)	340	14.8	36.2	0.0
-	cooked (57% lean - 43% fat)	465	19.7	42.2	0.0
	separable lean				
+	raw	164	21.1	8.2	0.0
+	broiled	224	30.2	10.5	0.0
	separable fat				
-	raw	777	4.2	84.1	0.0
	good grade				
-	raw (64% lean - 36% fat)	370	15.3	33.8	0.0
-	broiled (58%lean - 42% fat)	446	20.5	39.7	0.0
	separable lean				
-	raw	370	15.3	33.8	0.0
-	broiled	446	20.5	39.7	0.0
	separable fat				
-	raw	775	4.3	83.9	0.0
	T-Bone Steak				
	choice grade				
-	raw (62% lean - 38% fat)	397	14.7	37.1	0.0
-	broiled (56% lean - 44% fat)	473	19.5	43.2	0.0
	separable lean				
+	raw	164	21.2	8.1	0.0
+	broiled	223	30.4	10.3	0.0
	separable fat				
-	raw	774	4.3	83.8	0.0
*	Beet Greens, boiled	18	1.7	0.2	3.3
	Beverages				
	alcoholic				
*	beer	41	0.3	0.0	3.8
*	gin, vodka, whiskey (80 proof)	231	0.0	0.0	tr.
*	wine, dessert	137	0.0	0.0	7.7
*	wine, table	85	0.1	0.0	4.3

Standard Portion - 100 grams (3 1/2 ounces)				
food	**cal**	**pro gms**	**fat gms**	**carb gms**
non-alcohol				
* cola, carbonated	39	0.0	0.0	10.0
* cream soda	43	0.0	0.0	11.0
* fruit-flavor soda	46	0.0	0.0	12.0
* ginger ale	31	0.0	0.0	8.0
* root beer	41	0.0	0.0	10.5
Biscuit Dough				
- homemade	369	7.4	17.4	45.8
* commercial	277	7.3	6.4	46.4
Blackberries				
* canned, heavy syrup	91	0.8	0.6	22.2
Blackberry Juice				
* canned, unsweetened	37	0.3	0.6	7.8
Blueberries				
* raw	62	0.7	0.5	15.3
* frozen, unsweetened	55	0.7	0.5	13.6
* frozen, sweetened	105	0.6	0.3	26.5
+ Bluefish, broiled	159	26.2	5.2	0.0
* Boston brown bread	211	5.5	1.3	45.6
+ Bouillon Cubes	120	20.0	3.0	5.0
Boysenberries				
* frozen, unsweetened	48	1.2	0.3	11.4
* frozen, sweetened	96	0.8	0.3	24.4
- Brains, all kinds	125	10.4	8.6	0.8
* Bran	240	12.6	3.0	74.3
* Bran Flakes	303	10.2	1.8	80.6
* Bran Flakes w/raisins	287	8.3	1.4	79.3
- Brazilnuts	654	14.3	66.9	10.9
Breads				
* cracked wheat	263	8.6	2.2	52.1
* cracked wheat toasted	313	10.4	2.6	62.0
* raisin, plain	262	6.6	2.8	53.6
* rye, american	243	9.1	1.1	52.1
* rye, toasted	282	10.6	1.3	60.5

	Standard Portion - 100 grams (3 1/2 ounces)			
	food	**cal**	**pro gms**	**fat gms**	**carb gms**
	white, 4% milk				
*	plain	270	8.7	3.2	50.5
*	toasted	314	10.1	3.7	58.8
	whole wheat, 2% milk				
*	plain	243	10.5	3.0	47.7
*	toasted	289	12.5	3.6	56.7
*	Breadcrumbs, dry	392	12.6	4.6	73.4
*	Bread Pudding	187	5.6	6.1	28.4
	Bread Stuffing				
-	dry	358	6.5	21.8	35.6
-	moist	208	4.4	12.8	19.7
	Broccoli				
*	raw	32	3.6	0.3	5.9
*	boiled	26	3.1	0.3	4.5
	Brussel Sprouts				
*	raw	45	4.9	0.4	8.3
*	boiled	36	4.2	0.4	6.4
*	Buckwheat, whole-grain	335	11.7	2.4	72.9
*	Bulgur, hard red winter	354	11.2	1.5	75.7
+	Bullhead, black, raw	84	16.3	1.6	0.0
-	Butter	716	0.6	81.0	0.4
-	Butter, oil or dehydrated	876	0.3	99.5	0.0
+/-	Butterfish, raw	169	18.1	10.2	0.0
*	Buttermilk, cultured	36	3.6	0.1	5.1
-	Butternuts	629	23.7	61.2	8.4
	Cabbage				
*	raw	24	1.3	0.2	5.4
*	cooked	18	1.0	0.2	4.0
	Cakes, home recipes				
*	angelfood	269	7.1	0.2	60.2
-	chocolate w/icing	369	4.5	16.4	55.8
*/-	fruitcake, dark	379	4.8	15.3	59.7
*/-	gingerbread	317	3.8	10.7	52.0
-	pound, old fashioned	473	5.7	29.5	47.0
*	sponge, white w/out icing	375	4.6	16.0	54.0

Standard Portion - 100 grams (3 1/2 ounces)

	food	cal	pro gms	fat gms	carb gms
	Cakes, mix recipe				
*	coffeecake w/egg & milk	322	6.3	9.6	52.4
*	devil's food w/egg & icing	339	4.4	12.3	58.3
*	gingerbread w/water	276	3.1	6.8	51.1
*	white w/egg & icing	351	3.9	10.7	62.8
	Cake Icings				
*	caramel	360	1.3	6.7	76.5
*/-	chocolate	376	3.2	13.9	67.4
*	white	376	0.5	6.6	81.6
	Candy				
*	caramels	399	4.0	10.2	76.6
*	gumdrops	347	0.1	0.7	87.4
*	marshmallows	319	2.0	tr.	80.4
*/-	peanut brittle	421	5.7	10.4	81.0
	Chocolate				
-	bittersweet	507	4.2	35.7	57.0
*/-	fudge	400	2.7	12.2	75.0
*/-	fudge w/nuts	426	3.9	17.4	69.0
-	milk	520	7.7	32.3	56.9
	chocolate coated				
-	almonds	569	12.3	43.7	39.6
-	fudge w/caramel & peanuts	433	7.7	18.1	64.1
-	peanuts	561	16.4	41.3	39.1
*/-	raisins	425	5.4	17.1	70.5
+	Carp, raw	115	18.0	4.2	0.0
	Carrots				
*	raw	42	1.1	0.2	9.7
*	cooked, drained	31	0.9	0.2	7.1
*	canned, solids	30	0.8	0.3	6.7
-	Cashew Nuts	561	17.2	45.7	29.3
+	Catfish, raw	103	17.6	3.1	0.0
	Cauliflower				
*	raw	27	2.7	0.2	5.2
*	cooked, drained	22	2.3	0.2	4.1

Standard Portion - 100 grams (3 1/2 ounces)				
food	**cal**	**pro gms**	**fat gms**	**carb gms**
Caviar				
+/- sturgeon, granular	262	26.9	15.0	3.3
Celery				
* raw	17	0.9	0.1	3.9
* cooked, drained	14	0.8	0.1	3.1
Chard, Swiss				
* raw	25	2.4	0.3	4.6
* cooked, drained	18	1.8	0.2	3.3
Cheese				
- bleu, roquefort	368	21.5	30.5	2.0
- brick	299	17.5	24.7	1.8
Chicken				
chicken w/skin				
+ light meat, raw	120	19.9	3.9	0.0
+/- light meat, cooked	234	31.5	9.9	2.4
+/- light meat, fried	234	31.5	9.9	2.4
+/- dark meat, raw	132	17.7	6.3	0.0
+/- dark meat,cooked	263	29.9	13.6	3.1
+/- dark meat, fried	263	29.9	13.6	3.1
chicken w/out skin				
+ light meat, raw	117	23.4	1.9	0.0
+ light meat, cooked	166	31.5	3.4	0.0
+ light meat, roast	166	31.5	3.4	0.0
+ dark meat, raw	130	20.6	4.7	0.0
+ dark meat, cooked	176	28.0	6.3	0.0
+ dark meat, roast	176	28.0	6.3	0.0
+/- chicken, canned	198	21.6	11.7	0.0
- chicken & noodles	153	9.3	7.7	10.7
- potpie, frozen	219	6.7	11.5	22.2
- Chub, raw	145	15.3	8.8	7.1
* Citron, candied	314	0.2	0.3	80.2
+ Clams	76	12.6	1.6	2.0
- Clam Fritters	311	11.4	15.0	30.9

Standard Portion - 100 grams (3 1/2 ounces)

	food	cal	pro gms	fat gms	carb gms
	Cocoa Powder				
*	non-fat milk	359	18.6	2.0	70.8
*	hot chocolate mix	392	9.4	10.6	73.9
-	breakfast, high fat	299	16.8	23.7	48.3
-	breakfast, med. fat	220	19.2	12.7	53.8
	Coconut Meat				
-	fresh	346	3.5	35.3	9.4
-	dried, sweetened	548	3.6	39.1	53.2
+	Cod, broiled	170	28.4	5.3	0.0
*	Coffee	1	tr.	tr.	tr.
	Coleslaw				
-	w/french dressing	129	1.1	12.3	5.1
-	w/mayonnaise	95	1.3	14.0	4.8
	Collards				
*	raw w/out stem	45	4.8	0.8	7.5
*	boiled w/out stem	33	3.6	0.7	5.1
	Cookies				
-	brownies w/nuts	485	6.5	31.3	50.9
-	butter, thin & rich	457	6.1	16.9	70.9
-	chocolate chip	516	5.4	30.1	60.1
*	fig bars	358	3.9	5.6	75.4
*	gingersnaps	420	5.5	8.9	79.8
*/-	oatmeal w/raisins	451	6.2	15.4	73.5
-	peanut	473	10.0	19.1	67.0
-	shortbread	498	7.2	23.1	65.1
*/-	sugar	444	6.0	16.8	68.0
*/-	vanilla wafers	462	5.4	16.1	74.4
	Cookie Dough, plain				
-	unbaked	449	3.5	22.6	58.8
-	baked	469	3.9	25.0	64.9
	Corn, sweet				
*	white or yellow	96	3.5	1.0	22.1
*	kernels, on cob	91	3.3	1.0	21.0
*	canned, creamed	82	2.1	0.6	20.0
*	canned, whole	84	2.6	0.8	19.8

Standard Portion - 100 grams (3 1/2 ounces)

	food	cal	pro gms	fat gms	carb gms
	Corn Bread				
*	johnnycake	267	8.7	5.2	45.5
-	spoonbread	195	6.7	11.4	16.9
*	Corn Flour	368	7.8	2.6	76.8
-	Corn Fritters	377	7.8	21.5	39.7
*	Corn, puffed	399	8.1	4.2	80.8
*	Corn Pudding	104	4.0	4.7	13.0
	Cornmeal, white or yellow				
*	dry	364	7.9	1.2	78.4
*	cooked	50	1.1	0.2	10.7
*	Cornstarch	362	0.3	tr.	87.6
*	Cowpeas, boiled	127	9.0	0.8	21.8
	Crab				
+	steamed	93	17.3	1.9	0.5
+	canned	101	17.4	2.5	1.1
*	Crabapples, raw	68	0.4	0.3	17.8
	Crackers				
*	animal	429	6.6	9.4	79.9
-	cheese	479	11.2	21.3	60.4
*	graham, plain	384	8.0	9.4	73.3
*	saltines	433	8.0	12.0	71.5
*	soda	439	9.2	13.1	70.6
*/-	whole wheat	403	8.4	13.8	68.2
*	Cranberries, raw	46	0.4	0.7	10.8
*	Cranberry Juice	65	0.1	0.1	16.5
*	Cranberry Sauce	146	0.1	0.2	37.5
+	Crappie, white, raw	79	16.8	0.8	0.0
+	Crayfish, raw	72	14.6	0.5	1.2
	Cream, fluid				
-	half & half	134	3.2	11.7	4.6
-	heavy, whipping	352	2.2	37.6	3.1
-	Cream subsitutes, dry	508	8.5	26.7	61.3
-	Cream Puffs, custard	233	6.5	13.9	20.5
*	Cress, garden, raw	32	2.6	0.7	5.5

Standard Portion - 100 grams (3 1/2 ounces)

	food	cal	pro gms	fat gms	carb gms
+	Croaker, atlantic, baked	133	24.3	3.2	0.0
*	Cucumbers, raw	14	0.6	0.1	3.2
*	Currents, raw	54	1.7	0.1	13.1
*	Custard, baked	115	5.4	5.5	11.1
	Dandelion Greens				
*	raw	45	2.7	0.7	9.2
*	boiled	33	2.0	0.6	6.4
*	Dates, natural/dry	274	2.2	0.5	72.9
-	Dolly Varden, raw	144	19.9	6.5	0.0
	Doughnuts				
-	cake	391	4.6	18.6	51.4
-	yeast	414	6.3	26.7	37.7
	Duck, raw, flesh only				
-	domesticated	165	21.4	8.2	0.0
+	wild	138	21.3	5.2	0.0
-	Eclair, custard	239	6.2	13.6	23.2
-	Eel, raw	233	15.9	18.3	0.0
	Eggs				
-	raw, whole	163	12.9	11.5	0.9
+	raw, white	51	10.9	tr.	0.8
-	raw, yolk	348	16.0	30.6	0.6
-	cooked, fried	216	13.8	17.2	0.3
-	cooked, hard-boiled	163	12.9	11.5	0.9
-	cooked, omelet	173	11.2	12.9	2.4
-	cooked, poached	163	12.7	11.6	0.8
-	cooked, scrambled	173	11.2	12.9	2.4
*	Eggplant, cooked	19	1.0	0.2	4.1
-	Eulachon (smelt), raw	118	14.6	6.2	0.0
*	Farina, cooked	42	1.3	0.1	8.7
-	Fats, cooking	884	0.0	99.9	0.0
*	Fennel, raw leaves	28	2.8	0.4	5.1
	Figs				
*	canned, heavy syrup	84	0.5	0.2	16.8
*	dried, uncooked	274	4.3	1.3	69.1

Standard Portion - 100 grams (3 1/2 ounces)

	food	cal	pro gms	fat gms	carb gms
-	Filberts (hazelnuts)	634	12.6	62.4	16.7
+	Finnan Haddie (Haddock)	103	23.2	0.4	0.0
-	Fish cakes, frozen	270	9.2	17.9	17.2
-	Fish Sticks, frozen	176	16.6	8.9	6.5
+	Flatfishes, raw	79	16.7	0.8	0.0
+	Flounder, broiled	202	30.0	8.2	0.0
+	Frog Legs, raw	73	16.4	0.3	0.0
	Fruit Cocktail				
*	canned, water pack	37	0.4	0.1	9.7
*	canned, heavy syrup	76	0.4	0.1	19.7
*	Garlic, raw cloves	137	6.2	0.2	30.8
	Gelatin, dry				
*	desserts w/water	59	1.5	0.0	14.1
*	desserts w/fruit	67	1.3	0.1	16.4
*	Ginger Root, fresh	49	1.4	1.0	9.5
+	Gizzard, chicken, cooked	148	27.0	3.3	0.7
	Goose, domesticated				
-	flesh/skin, raw	371	15.9	33.6	0.0
-	flesh/skin, cooked	441	22.9	38.1	0.0
+	flesh only, raw	159	22.3	7.1	0.0
+	flesh only, cooked	233	33.9	9.8	0.0
	Gooseberries				
*	canned, heavy syrup	90	0.5	0.1	23.0
*	fresh	39	0.8	0.2	9.7
	Grapefruit				
*	all kinks, raw	41	0.5	0.1	10.6
*	juice, all kinds	39	0.5	0.1	9.2
*	canned, water	30	0.6	0.1	17.8
*	canned, syrup	70	0.6	0.1	17.8
*	frozen juice/water	41	0.5	0.1	9.8
*	Grapes, raw	69	1.3	1.0	15.7
	Grape Juice				
*	canned/bottled	66	0.2	tr.	16.6
*	frozen/water	53	0.2	tr.	13.3

Standard Portion - 100 grams (3 1/2 ounces)				
food	cal	pro gms	fat gms	carb gms
* Guavas, whole, raw	62	0.8	0.6	15.0
+ Guinea Hen, raw	158	23.4	6.4	0.0
Haddock				
+ raw	79	18.3	0.1	0.0
+/- fried	165	19.6	6.4	5.8
Halibut				
+ raw	100	20.9	1.2	0.0
+ broiled	171	25.2	7.0	0.0
+ Heart, braised	188	31.3	5.7	0.7
Herring				
+/- atlantic, poached	176	17.3	11.3	0.0
+ pacific, poached	98	17.5	2.6	0.0
- Hickorynuts	673	13.2	68.7	12.8
* Honey	304	0.3	0.0	82.3
* Horseradish, prepared	38	1.3	0.2	9.6
Ice Cream				
- 10% fat	192	4.5	10.6	20.8
- 12% fat	207	4.0	12.5	20.6
- 16% fat	222	2.6	16.1	18.0
* Ice Cream Cone	377	10.0	2.4	77.9
* Ice Milk	152	4.8	5.1	22.4
+ Jack Mackerel, raw	143	21.6	5.6	0.0
* Jams & Preserves	272	0.6	0.1	70.0
* Jellies	273	0.1	0.1	70.6
* Kale, cooked, no stems	39	4.5	0.7	6.1
- Kidneys, braised	252	33.0	12.0	0.8
+ Kingfish, raw	105	18.3	3.0	0.0
* Kumquats, raw	65	0.9	0.1	17.1
+ Lake Herring, raw	96	17.7	2.3	0.0
+/- Lake Trout, raw	168	18.3	10.0	0.0
Lamb				
- leg, roasted	279	25.3	18.9	0.0
- loin, roasted	359	22.0	29.4	0.0
- Lard	902	0.0	99.9	0.0
* Leeks, raw	52	2.2	0.3	11.2

Standard Portion - 100 grams (3 1/2 ounces)

	food	cal	pro gms	fat gms	carb gms
*	Lemons	20	1.2	0.3	10.7
	Lemon Juice				
*	fresh	25	0.5	0.2	8.0
*	frozen, unsweetened	22	0.4	0.2	7.2
*	Lemonade w/water	44	0.1	tr.	11.4
*	Lentils, cooked	106	7.8	tr.	19.3
	Lettuce				
*	raw, iceberg	13	0.9	0.1	2.9
*	raw, looseleaf	18	1.3	0.3	3.5
*	Limes, raw	28	0.7	0.2	9.5
*	Lime juice, unsweetened	26	0.3	0.1	9.0
+	Lincod, raw	84	17.9	0.8	0.0
+	Liver, beef, fried	165	26.5	4.4	3.1
+	Lobster, raw	91	16.9	1.9	0.5
+/-	Lobster Newburg	194	18.5	10.6	5.1
	Loganberries				
*	raw	62	1.0	0.6	14.9
*	canned, heavy syrup	89	0.6	0.4	22.2
+	Lungs, beef, raw	96	17.6	2.3	0.0
	Lychees				
*	raw	64	0.9	0.3	16.4
*	dried	277	3.8	1.2	70.7
-	Macademia Nuts	691	7.8	71.6	15.9
*	Macaroni, cooked	111	3.4	0.4	23.0
	Macaroni & Cheese				
*/-	canned	95	3.9	4.0	10.7
*/-	home recipe	215	8.4	11.1	20.1
	Mackerel, atlantic				
-	raw	191	19.0	12.2	0.0
-	broiled	236	21.8	15.8	0.0
-	smoked	219	23.8	13.0	0.0
*	Malt, dry	368	13.1	1.9	77.4
*	Malt Extract, dry	367	6.0	tr.	89.2
*	Mangos, raw	66	0.7	0.4	16.8

Standard Portion - 100 grams (3 1/2 oounces)				
food	**cal**	**pro gms**	**fat gms**	**carb gms**
- Margarine	720	0.6	81.0	0.4
* Marmalade, citrus	257	0.5	0.1	70.1
- Mayonaise	720	0.6	81.0	0.4
Milk, cow				
- whole 3.7%	66	3.5	3.7	4.9
+/* skim	36	3.6	0.1	5.1
+/* partly skimmed 2%	59	4.2	2.0	6.0
- canned, evaporated	137	7.0	7.9	9.7
* canned, condensed	321	8.1	8.7	54.3
- dry, whole	502	26.4	27.5	38.2
+/* dry, skim, instant	359	35.8	0.7	51.6
- chocolate, whole	85	3.4	3.4	11.0
- Milk, goat	67	3.2	4.0	4.6
- Milk, human	77	1.1	4.0	4.6
- Milk, reindeer	234	10.8	19.6	4.1
* Molasses, cane	232	0.0	0.0	60.0
Muffins				
*/- plain, home recipe	294	7.8	10.1	42.3
*/- blueberry, home recipe	281	7.3	9.3	41.9
*/- bran, home recipe	261	7.7	9.8	43.1
*/- mixes w/egg, milk	324	6.0	10.6	50.0
*/- mixes w/egg, water	297	4.5	7.8	51.9
+ Mullet, striped, raw	146	19.6	6.9	0.0
* Mushrooms, raw	28	2.7	0.3	4.4
Muskmellons, raw				
* cantaloup	30	0.7	0.1	7.5
* casaba	27	1.2	tr.	6.5
* honeydew	33	0.8	0.3	7.7
+ Mussels, meat only	95	14.4	2.2	3.3
Mustard Greens				
* raw	31	3.0	0.5	5.6
* cooked	23	2.2	0.4	4.0
Mustard, prepared				
- brown	91	5.9	6.3	5.3
* yellow	75	4.7	4.4	6.4

Standard Portion - 100 grams (3 1/2 oounces)				
food	**cal**	**pro gms**	**fat gms**	**carb gms**
* Nectarines,raw	64	0.6	tr.	17.1
New Zealand Spinach				
* raw	19	2.2	0.3	3.1
* cooked	13	1.7	0.2	2.1
- Noodles, chow mein	489	13.2	23.5	58.0
* Noodles, egg	125	4.1	1.5	23.3
Oatmeal/rolled oats				
* dry	390	14.2	7.4	68.2
* cooked	55	2.0	1.0	9.7
Ocean Perch, atlantic				
+ raw or poached	88	18.0	1.2	0.0
- fried	227	19.0	13.3	6.8
+ Octopus, raw	73	15.3	0.8	0.0
- Oils, salad/cooking	884	0.0	99.9	0.0
Okra				
* raw	36	2.4	0.3	7.6
* cooked	29	2.2	0.3	6.0
Olives				
- green	116	1.4	12.7	1.3
- ripe, manzanilla	129	1.1	13.8	2.6
- ripe, greek style	338	2.2	35.8	8.7
Onions				
* raw	38	1.5	0.1	8.7
* young green, raw	36	1.5	0.2	8.2
+/- Opossum, roasted	221	30.2	10.2	0.0
* Oranges, raw	49	1.0	0.2	12.2
Orange Juice				
* raw, commercial	45	0.7	0.2	10.4
* canned, unsweetened	48	0.8	0.2	11.2
* frozen, diluted	45	0.7	0.1	10.7
Oysters				
+ raw, meat only	91	10.6	2.2	6.4
- fried	239	8.6	13.9	18.6
Oyster Stew				
- frozen w/milk	84	4.2	4.9	5.9
- home recipe w/milk	97	5.2	6.4	4.5

Standard Portion - 100 grams (3 1/2 ounces)				
food	**cal**	**pro gms**	**fat gms**	**carb gms**
Pancakes				
*/- home recipe	231	7.1	7.0	34.1
*/- dry, w/egg & milk	225	7.2	7.3	32.4
* Papayas, raw	39	0.6	0.1	10.0
* Parsley, common	44	3.6	0.6	8.5
Parsnips				
* raw	76	1.7	0.5	17.5
* cooked	66	1.5	0.5	14.9
Peaches				
* raw	38	0.6	0.1	9.7
* canned, heavy syrup	78	0.4	0.1	20.1
* dehydrated, uncooked	340	4.8	0.9	88.0
* Peach Nectar, canned	48	0.2	tr.	12.4
Peanuts				
- raw, with skins	564	26.0	47.5	18.6
- roasted & salted	585	26.0	49.8	18.8
- Peanut Butter	581	27.8	49.4	17.2
Pears				
* raw	61	0.7	0.4	15.3
* canned, heavy syrup	76	0.2	0.2	19.6
* dried, uncooked	268	3.1	1.8	67.3
* Pear Nectar, canned	52	0.3	0.2	13.2
Peas				
* green, raw	84	6.3	0.4	14.4
* green, canned	88	4.7	0.4	16.8
* green, cooked	71	5.4	0.4	12.1
* green, frozen	68	5.1	0.3	11.8
* podded, raw	84	6.3	0.4	14.4
* podded, cooked	43	2.9	9.2	9.5
- Pecans	687	9.2	71.2	14.6
Peppers, hot				
* raw, green	37	1.3	0.2	9.1
* raw, red	93	3.7	2.3	18.1
* dried, chili powder	340	14.3	12.4	56.5

Standard Portion - 100 grams (3 1/2 ounces)				
food	cal	pro gms	fat gms	carb gms
Peppers, sweet				
* green, raw	22	1.2	0.2	4.8
* red, raw	31	1.4	0.3	7.1
Perch, raw				
+ white	118	19.3	4.0	0.0
+ yellow	91	19.5	0.9	0.0
* Persimmons, raw	127	0.8	0.4	33.5
+ Pheasant, flesh only, raw	139	20.8	4.9	1.6
Pickles				
* cucumbers, dill	11	0.7	0.2	2.2
* cucumbers, sweet	146	0.7	0.4	36.5
* chowchow, sweet	116	1.5	0.9	29.7
* relish, sweet	138	0.5	0.6	34.0
Pies				
- apple	256	2.2	11.1	38.1
- banana cream	221	4.5	9.3	30.7
- blackberry	243	2.6	11.0	34.4
- cherry	261	2.6	11.3	38.4
- chocolate chiffon	328	6.8	15.3	43.7
- custard	218	6.1	11.1	23.4
- lemon meringue	255	3.7	10.2	37.7
- mince	271	2.5	11.5	41.2
- pecan	418	5.1	22.9	51.3
- pumpkin	211	4.0	11.2	24.5
- rhubarb	253	2.5	10.7	38.2
- strawberry	198	1.9	7.9	30.9
- sweet potato	213	4.5	11.3	23.7
- Piecrust, enriched flour	500	6.1	33.4	43.8
Piecrust Mix				
- dry form	522	7.2	32.7	49.5
- prepared w/water	464	6.4	29.1	44.0
- Pigs' Feet, pickled	199	16.7	14.8	0.0
* Pimentos, canned	27	0.9	0.5	5.8

Standard Portion - 100 grams (3 1/2 ounces)				
food	**cal**	**pro gms**	**fat gms**	**carb gms**
Pineapple				
* raw	52	0.4	0.2	13.7
* canned, juice pack	58	0.4	0.1	15.1
* canned, heavy syrup	74	0.3	0.1	19.4
* Pineapple Juice, canned	55	0.4	0.1	13.5
* Pineapple/Grapefruit Juice, canned	54	0.2	tr.	13.5
- Pinenuts	552	31.1	47.4	11.6
- Pistachio Nuts	594	19.3	53.7	19.0
Pizza w/ cheese				
- homemade	236	12.0	8.3	28.3
- homemade w/sausage	234	7.8	9.3	29.6
Plums				
* raw	66	0.5	tr.	17.8
* canned, heavy syrup	83	0.4	0.1	21.6
- Pompano, raw	166	18.8	9.5	0.0
Popcorn				
* plain	386	12.7	5.0	76.7
- oil & salt	456	9.8	21.8	59.7
* carmel	383	6.1	3.5	85.4
- Popovers, homemade	224	8.8	9.2	25.8
Pork				
- ham	374	23.0	30.6	0.0
- loin, roasted	362	24.5	28.5	0.0
- spareribs, braised	440	20.8	38.9	0.0
Potatoes				
* baked in skin	93	2.6	0.1	21.1
* boiled in skin	76	2.1	0.1	17.1
- french fries, fresh	274	4.3	13.2	36.0
- french fries, frozen	220	3.6	8.4	33.7
- fried from raw	268	4.0	14.2	32.6
- hash-browns, fresh	229	3.1	11.7	29.1
- hash-browns, frozen	224	2.0	1154	29.0
*/- mashed w/milk	94	2.1	4.3	12.3
* raw	76	2.1	0.1	17.1
- scalloped w/cheese	145	5.3	7.9	13.6

Standard Portion - 100 grams (3 1/2 ounces)

	food	cal	pro gms	fat gms	carb gms
-	Potato Chips	568	5.3	39.8	50.0
*	Potato Flour	351	8.0	0.8	79.9
-	Potato Salad, homemade	145	3.0	9.2	13.4
-	Potato Sticks	544	6.4	36.4	50.8
*	Pretzels	390	9.8	4.5	75.9
*	Prunes, dried	255	2.1	0.6	67.4
*	Prune Juice, canned/bottled	77	0.4	0.1	19.0
*	Prune Whip	156	4.4	0.2	36.9
	Puddings, homemade				
*/-	chocolate	148	3.1	4.7	25.7
*/-	vanilla	111	3.5	3.9	15.9
	Pumpkin				
*	raw	26	1.0	0.1	6.5
*	canned	33	1.0	0.3	7.9
-	Pumpkin/Squash Seeds, dry	553	29.0	46.7	15.0
+	Quail, w/ skin	172	25.4	7.0	0.0
+	Rabbit, flesh only	216	29.3	10.1	0.0
+/-	Racoon, roasted	255	29.2	14.5	0.0
*	Radishes, raw	17	1.0	0.1	3.6
*	Raisins, uncooked	289	2.5	0.2	77.4
	Raspberries				
*	raw, red	57	1.2	0.5	13.6
*	frozen, red	98	0.7	0.2	24.6
+	Red & Gray Snapper, raw	93	19.8	0.9	0.0
	Rhubarb				
*	raw	16	0.6	0.1	3.7
*	cooked w/sugar	141	0.5	0.1	36.0
	Rice				
*/-	bran	276	13.3	15.8	50.8
*	brown, cooked	119	2.5	0.6	25.5
*	flakes	390	5.9	0.3	87.7
*/-	polished	265	12.1	12.8	57.7
*	pudding w/raisins	146	3.6	3.1	26.7
*	puffed	399	6.0	0.4	89.5
*	white, cooked	109	2.0	0.1	24.2

	Standard Portion - 100 grams (3 1/2 ounces)				
	food	**cal**	**pro gms**	**fat gms**	**carb gms**
+	Rock Fish, steamed	107	18.1	2.5	1.9
	Rolls & Buns				
*	commercial, hard	312	9.8	3.2	59.5
*	commercial, plain	298	8.2	5.6	53,9
*	commercial, sweet	316	8.5	9.1	49.3
*	commercial, whole wheat	257	10.0	2.8	52.3
*	homemade w/milk	339	8.2	8.7	56.1
	Rutabagas, boiled	35	0.9	0.1	8.2
*	Rye Flour	350	11.4	1.7	74.8
*	Rye Wafers	344	13.0	1.2	76.3
-	Sablefish, raw	190	13.0	14.9	0.0
	Salad Dressings				
	low-fat				
-	bleu cheese, roquefort	76	3.0	5.9	4.1
*/-	french	96	0.4	4.3	15.6
	regular				
-	bleu cheese, roquefort	504	4.8	52.3	7.4
-	french	410	0.6	38.9	17.5
-	italian	552	0.2	60.0	6.9
-	thousand island	502	0.8	50.2	15.4
	Salmon, atlantic				
+/-	canned	203	21.7	12.2	0.0
+	baked	182	27.0	7.4	0.0
+/-	smoked	176	21.6	9.3	0.0
*	Salt Sticks	384	12.0	2.9	75.3
-	Sandwich Spread	379	0.7	36.2	15.9
	Sardines				
-	canned in oil	203	24.0	11.1	0.0
-	canned in brine	196	18.8	12.0	1.7
-	canned in tomato	197	18.7	12.2	1.7
*	Sauerkraut	18	1.0	0.2	4.0

Standard Portion - 100 grams (3 1/2 ounoces)

	food	cal	pro gms	fat gms	carb gms
	Sausage, cold cuts				
-	blood sausage	394	14.1	36.9	0.3
-	bologna	304	12.1	27.5	1.1
-	braunschweiger	319	14.8	27.4	2.3
-	brown & serve	422	16.5	37.8	2.8
-	country sausage	345	15.1	31.1	0.0
-	deviled ham, canned	351	13.9	32.3	0.0
-	frankfurters	304	12.4	27.2	1.6
-	headcheese	268	15.5	22.0	1.0
-	knockwurst	278	14.1	23.2	2.2
-	liverwurst, fresh	307	16.2	25.6	1.8
-	lunch meat, ham	234	19.0	17.0	0.0
-	lunch meat, pork	294	15.0	24.9	1.3
-	meat loaf	200	15.9	13.2	3.3
-	meat, potted	248	17.5	19.2	0.0
-	polish sausage	304	15.7	25.8	1.2
-	pork sausage	476	18.1	44.2	tr.
-	salami, dry	450	23.8	38.1	1.2
-	vienna sausage	240	14.0	19.8	0.3
	Scallops, bay & sea				
+/-	fried, breaded	194	18.0	8.4	10.5
+	steamed	112	23.2	1.4	tr.
+	Seabass, white, raw	96	21.4	0.5	0.0
-	Seaweed, kelp, raw	0	0.0	1.1	0.0
-	Sesame Seeds, dry	582	18.2	53.4	17.6
+/-	Shad, baked	201	23.2	11.3	0.0
+	Sheepshead, atlantic, raw	113	20.6	2.8	0.0
*	Sherbet, orange	134	0.9	1.2	30.8
	Shrimp				
+	raw	91	18.1	0.8	1.5
+/-	fried	225	20.3	10.8	10.0
+	canned	80	16.2	0.8	0.8
+	Shrimp/Lobster Paste	180	20.8	9.4	1.5

Standard Portion - 100 grams (3 1/2 ounces)				
food	**cal**	**pro gms**	**fat gms**	**carb gms**
Syrup				
* cane	263	0.0	0.0	68.0
* maple	252	0.0	0.0	65.0
* sorghum	257	0.0	0.0	68.0
* corn, light/dark	290	0.0	0.0	75.0
+ Skate, raw	98	21.5	0.7	0.0
+ Snail, raw	90	16.1	1.4	2.0
Soup - refer to can label				
Soybean, immature seeds				
+/- canned	103	9.0	5.0	7.4
*/- cooked	118	9.8	5.1	10.1
* miso, cereal	171	10.5	4.6	23.5
+/- Soybean Curd (tofu)	72	7.8	4.2	2.4
Soybean Four				
+/* defatted	326	47.0	0.9	38.1
- full-fat	421	36.7	20.3	30.4
Soybean Milk				
- fluid	33	3.4	1.5	2.2
- powder	429	41.8	20.3	28.0
* Soy Sauce	68	5.6	1.3	9.5
* Spagetti, cooked	111	3.4	0.4	23.0
Spinach				
* raw	26	3.2	0.3	4.3
* cooked	23	3.0	0.3	3.6
+ Spleen, raw	104	18.1	3.0	0.0
Squab				
- flesh w/skin, raw	294	18.5	23.8	0.0
+/- flesh only, raw	142	17.5	7.5	0.0
Squash				
* summer, raw	19	1.1	0.1	4.2
* summer, boiled	14	0.9	0.1	3.1
* winter, raw	50	1.4	0.3	12.4
* winter, cooked	38	1.1	0.3	9.2
+ Squid, raw	84	16.4	0.9	1.5

Standard Portion - 100 grams (3 1/2 ounces)

	food	cal	pro gms	fat gms	carb gms
*	Strawberries, raw	37	0.7	0.5	8.4
+	Sturgeon, steamed	160	25.4	5.7	0.0
*	Succotash, thawed	93	4.2	0.4	20.5
-	Suet, raw	854	1.5	94.0	0.0
	Sugar				
*	beet/cane, brown	373	0.0	0.0	96.4
*	beet/cane, powder	385	0.0	0.0	99.5
*	beet/cane, white	385	0.0	0.0	99.5
*	maple	348	0.0	0.0	90.0
	Sweetbread				
-	beef, braised	320	25.9	23.2	0.0
+	calf, braised	168	32.5	3.2	0.0
+	lamb, braised	175	28.1	6.1	0.0
	Sweet Potatoes				
*	raw	114	1.7	0.4	26.3
*	baked in skin	141	2.1	0.5	32.5
*	candied	168	1.3	3.3	34.2
*	canned w/syrup	114	1.0	0.2	27.5
+	Swordfish, broiled	174	28.0	6.0	0.0
*	Tangerines, raw	46	0.8	0.2	11.6
*/-	Tapioca Pudding	134	5.0	5.1	17.1
-	Tartar Sauce	531	1.4	57.8	4.2
*	Tea	2	0.0	tr.	0.4
+	Tilefish, baked	138	24.5	3.7	0.0
	Tomatoes				
*	green, raw	24	1.2	0.2	5.1
*	red, raw	22	1.1	0.2	4.7
*	canned	21	1.0	0.2	4.3
*	Tomato Catsup	106	2.0	0.4	25.4
*	Tomato Chili Sauce	104	2.5	0.3	24.8
*	Tomato Juice, canned	19	0.9	0.1	4.3
*	Tomato Juice Cocktail	21	0.7	0.1	5.0
*	Tomato Paste, canned	82	3.4	0.4	18.6
*	Tomato Puree, canned	39	1.7	0.2	8.9

	Standard Portion - 100 grams (3 1/2 ounces)				
	food	**cal**	**pro gms**	**fat gms**	**carb gms**
	Tomcod, atlantic, raw	77	17.2	0.4	0.0
-	Tongue, beef, cooked	244	21.5	16.7	0.4
+	Tripe, beef	100	19.1	2.0	0.0
	Trout				
+	brook, raw	101	19.2	2.1	0.0
+/-	rainbow, raw	195	21.5	11.4	0.0
	Tuna				
+	yellow fin, poached	332	4.7	3.0	0.0
+/-	canned, oil	197	28.8	8.2	0.0
+	canned, water	127	28.0	0.8	0.0
	Turkey				
+	light meat w/out skin	176	32.9	3.9	0.0
+/-	canned, meat only	202	20.9	12.5	0.0
	Turnips				
*	raw	30	1.0	0.2	6.6
*	boiled	23	0.8	0.2	4.9
	Turnip Greens				
*	raw	28	3.0	0.3	5.0
*	boiled	20	2.2	0.2	3.6
+	Turtle, green, canned	106	23.4	0.6	0.0
+/-	Veal, loin	234	26.4	13.4	0.0
*	Vegetable Juice, canned	17	0.9	0.1	3.6
*	Vegetables, mixed, frozen	64	3.2	0.3	13.4
+	Venison, raw	126	21.0	4.0	0.0
	Vinegar				
*	cider	14	tr.	0.0	5.9
*	distilled	12	0.0	0.0	5.0
*	Waffles, frozen	253	7.1	6.2	42.0
-	Walnuts, english	651	14.8	64.0	15.8
*	Water Chestnut, raw	79	1.4	0.2	19.0
*	Watercress, raw	19	2.2	0.3	3.0
*	Watermelon, raw	26	0.5	0.2	6.4
+/-	Weakfish, broiled	208	24.6	11.4	0.0
-	Welch Rarebit	179	8.1	13.6	6.3

Standard Portion - 100 grams (3 1/2 ounces)

	food	cal	pro gms	fat gms	carb gms
*	Wheat, whole grain	330	12.3	1.8	71.7
*	Wheat Flour, whole	333	13.2	2.0	71.0
*	Wheat Bran	213	15.0	4.6	61.9
*/-	Wheat Germ	363	26.6	10.9	46.7
	Wheat Products				
*	cereal, cooked	75	2.2	0.4	16.9
*	cereal flakes	354	10.2	0.6	80.5
*	cereal, instant	80	3.0	0.3	16.1
*/-	Wheat Germ, toasted	391	30.0	11.5	49.5
*	Wheat, puffed	363	15.0	1.5	78.5
*	Wheat, shredded	354	9.9	2.0	78.9
*	Whey, dried	349	12.9	1.1	73.5
	Whitefish, lake				
-	baked, stuffed	215	15.2	14.0	5.8
+/-	raw	155	18.9	8.2	0.0
+/-	smoked	155	20.9	7.3	0.0
-	White Sauce	162	3.9	12.5	8.8
*	Wild Rice, raw	353	14.1	0.7	75.3
*	Yam, raw	101	2.1	0.2	23.2
	Yeast				
*	dry, active	282	35.9	1.6	38.9
*	brewers, debitter	283	38.8	1.0	38.4
	Yogurt				
*/+	low fat milk	50	3.4	1.7	5.2
*/-	whole milk	62	3.0	3.4	4.9
*	Zwieback	423	10.7	8.8	74.3

Appendix 2

Reference

The portion of our food table is a condensed version of *Composition of Foods* by Bernice K. Watt and Annabel L. Merril. Our work refers only to the calories, protein, fat, and carbohydrate content. *Composition of Foods* is the most comprehensive and thorough book of its kind. The mineral, fiber, and some vitamin content is recorded. All foods are listed in 3 1/2 ounces or 100 grams portions. This book is a most valuable resources.

Obtaining A Body Composition

A place to begin searching for a body composition evaluation would be your local health clubs. Staff and trainers are often available to make the evaluation or guide you in the right direction. If you do not have luck there, contact the athletic or exercise physiology department at a university in your area. Hospitals and health maintenance organizations are also offering this service in some communities.

If you are still stuck, call or write the distributor of the body compostion units themselves. Find out if they are aware of anyone in your area operating a unit. The companies listed can be contacted for additonal assistance and purchasing information.

Spectroscopy Units:

Fitness Analysis Computer Technology
6701 West 110 St.
Minneapolis, MN 55438
1-800-445-8418

Impedience Units:

RJL Systems Inc.
9930 Whittier
Detroit, MI 48224
1-800-528-4513

Cookbooks:

The American Heart Association Cookbook, 4th ed., Ballantine Books, 1984.

Grundy, Scott and Mary Winston, ed. *The American Heart Association Low Fat, Low Cholesterol Cookbook*, Times Books, 1989.

Hinman, Bobbie and Millie Snyder. *Lean & Luscious*, Prima Publishing, 1987.

Hinman, Bobbie and Millie Snyder. *More Lean & Luscious*, Prima Publishing, 1988.

Lappe, Frances M. *Diet for a Small Planet*, 10th anniversary ed., Ballantine Books, 1982.

Piscatella, Joseph. *Choices for a Healthy Heart*, Workman Publishing, 1987.

Piscatella, Joseph. *Don't Eat Your Heart Out*, Workman Publishing, 1987.

Shriver, Brenda and Ann Tinsley. *No Red Meat*, Fisher Books, 1989.

Weight Watchers Favorite Recipes, NAL Penguin, 1986.

Weight Watchers Quick and Easy Menu Cookbook, NAL Penguin, 1987.

Health

Bailey, Covert. *Fit or Fat?*, Houghton Mifflin, 1978.

Bland, Jeffery. *Assess Your Own Nutritient Status*, Keats, 1987.

Bland, Jeffery. *Your Health Under Seige*, Greene, 1982.

Cheraskin, E, et al. *Diet and Disease*, Keats, 1987.

Cleave, T.L. *The Saccharine Disease: The Master of Our Time*, Keats, 1975.

Connor, Sonia L. and William E. *New American Diet*, Simon & Schuster, 1989.

Katch, Frank and William McArdle. *Nutrition, Weight Control and Exercise*, 3rd ed., Lea & Febiger, 1988.

Katch, Frank. *Sports, Health and Nutrition,* Human Kinetics, 1986.

Kugler, Hans. *The Disease of Aging*, Keats, 1984.

McArdle, William, et. al. *Exercise Physiology: Energy, Nutrition & Human Performance*, Lea & Febiger, 1986.

Robbins, John. *Diet for a New America*, Stillpoint Publishing, 1987.

Sharkey, Brian. *Physiology of Fitness*, 2nd ed., Human Kinetics, 1984.

Smith, Lendon,M.D. *Foods for Healthy Kids*, Berkley Publishing, 1987.

Travell, Janet and David Simmons. *Myofascial Pain and Dysfunction: The Trigger Point Manual*, Williams and Wilkins, 1983.

Exercise Physiology and Training:

Astrand, Per-Olof, et al. *Textbook of Work Physiology*, 3rd ed. McGraw-Hill, 1986.

LaLanne, Elaine and Richard Benyo. *Fitness After Fifty: Elaine LaLanne's Complete Fitness Program*, Greene, 1986.

Pearl, Bill and Gary Moran. *Getting Stronger: Weight Training For Men and Women*, Shelter Publishing, 1988.

Pollock, Wilmore and Fox. *Exercise in Health and Disease*, Saunders, 1984.

Additional Reading:

Crumm, Thomas, *The Magic of Conflict: Turning a Life Into a Work of Art*, Simon and Shuster, 1988.

Dyer, Wayne, *Pulling Your Own Strings*, Avon, 1979.

Dyer, Wayne, *Your Erroneous Zones*, Avon 1977.

Gallwey, Timothy, *The Inner Game of Golf*, Random House, 1981.

Gallwey, Timothy, *Inner Tennis: Playing the Game*, Random House, 1976.

Robbins, Anthony, *Unlimited Power*, Fawcett, 1987.

About The Author

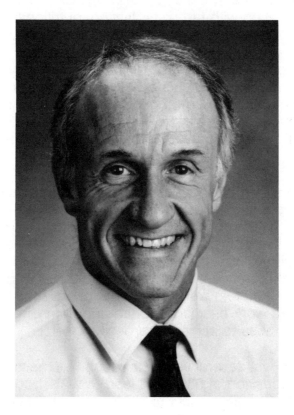

The research contributing to the Lean Body Promise grew out of a curiosity and desire to make changes in his own body. Dr. Quas describes his "former body" as broad in the middle with narrow shoulders and scrawny legs. His "slouched" posture was habit as years of practicing orthodontics took its toll. As a skier and beginning runner, Dr. Quas felt age bringing on more frequent and bothersome injuries, which often lingered for months. Refusing to accept the belief "this is what it means to grow older", Dr. Quas made a commitment to discover what worked to improve health, appearance, performance, and energy levels, and to communicate that message to those interested in changing their body.

In 1980, at age 40, Dr. Quas opened a center which provided body composition and fitness evaluations through hydrostatic testing. Clients enrolled in seminars to discuss food and training programs. Dr. Quas' earlier experimentation with fad diets, fasting, nutritional supplements and "health foods", mimmicked those attempts of his clients seeking positive, lasting changes. The body composition evaluations provided the opportunity to monitor and test the effects of a variety of diet programs and training activities. *The Lean Body Pomise* is the distillation of those tests. It is the shockingly honest answer to the questions we all have about weight and shape control.

Dr. Quas, an orthodontist, is trained to look at a patient and see the possibilities for improved appearance, health and function. Treatment takes time, based on the biologic limits of the body, as well as, the responsibility of patients to be active participants committed to the process. These same principles apply when making a change in weight and shape: patience to allow the body to work as it is designed and commitment to do what it takes to achieve the desired results.

For the last several years Dr. Quas has maintained a body composition of 93%-96% lean (4%-7% body fat) and coached many others to achieve and maintain the changes they want. His curiosity and commitment to excellence initiated this project, and is the fuel that drives him to discover "what's possible", in the area of human potential. This learning is ongoing through seminars and private coaching conducted by Dr. Quas and his staff in Bend, Oregon.

ORDER FORM

The Lean Body Promise:
Your Future Body an Owner's Manual $15.95

Quantity   _____
Subtotal   _____
SHIPPING - add $2.00 for the
first book, $.75 each addt'l   _____
TOTAL   _____

Name:_____

Address:_____

City:_____ State:_____ Zip:_____

Daytime telephone: (   ) _____

Mail this order form and a check or money order
for the total to:

SYNESIS PRESS
P.O. Box 1843-P, Bend, OR 97709

_____ I can't wait 3 - 4 weeks for Book Rate.
Here is $3.00 per book for Air Mail.

_____ Please send me information on the author's
Personal Development Seminar Series.

To order by phone, please call (503) 382-6517
FAX   (503) 382-0750